# Creating Well-Being for Couples and Families

*Increasing Health, Spirituality, and Happiness*

Susanne M. Alexander

***Creating Well-Being for Couples and Families***
ISBN: 978-1-940062-09-9
Published by Marriage Transformation LLC
United States of America
www.marriagetransformation.com

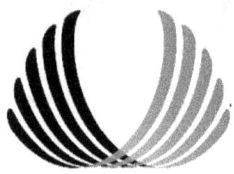

© 2020 Marriage Transformation LLC, all international rights reserved

No part of this book may be electronically shared, scanned or uploaded, or reproduced by any means, without the written permission of the publisher. Violations are theft of the author and publisher's intellectual property. *Thank you for respecting this legal copyright. Your integrity with this spreads a spirit of loving respect throughout the world and makes us very happy.*

This publication provides helpful and educational information about relationships. If expert assistance is required, the services of a competent professional should be sought. The examples and stories included are fictional or composites from the experience of couples shared with the author to maintain confidentiality.

**Cover Design Credit:** Steiner Graphics

**Cover Photographer:** McKinsey L. Jordan

**Layout:** Marriage Transformation

**Note:** Marriage Transformation® is a registered trademark in the United States. The logo of two wings of a bird symbolizing two partners in a relationship or marriage, both in color and in black and white, is copyrighted by Marriage Transformation.

*Creating Well-Being for Couples and Families*

## Dedication

*To my husband, Phil, who consistently encourages all aspects of my well-being. Thank you!*

*Creating Well-Being for Couples and Families*

## TABLE OF CONTENTS

Using This Guide

Getting Started

1. Character
2. Exercise
3. Nutrition
4. Relaxation
5. Sleep
6. Illness
7. Time
8. Friendship
9. Dates
10. Cleanliness
11. Sex
12. Parenting
13. Family
14. Work
15. Money

16. Communication
17. Listening
18. Appreciation
19. Feelings
20. Decisions
21. Humor
22. Nature
23. Creativity
24. Resilience
25. Resourcefulness
26. Spirituality
27. Service
28. Unity

Goal Setting

About the Author
About the Bahá'í Faith
Acknowledgements
Footnotes

## USING THIS GUIDE

Your commitment as a couple to your individual well-being, that of each other, your relationship or marriage, and your family empowers you to engage in constructive actions.

This guide will expand your perspectives on facets of well-being, providing a "tune-up" for some people and more ideas for others where this is a new concept. It will also focus you on ways to maintain and enhance well-being of all types, particularly for you as a couple.

Decades of science about couples seems to indicate that you can help each other become or stay healthier than individuals tend to be on their own. This book also includes a small selection of spiritual quotations drawn from the teachings of the Bahá'í Faith (www.bahai.org). Its teachings include the harmony of science and religion, and so both are included throughout. These teachings share this quotation about well-being for couples:

"And when He [God] desired to manifest grace and beneficence to men, and to set the world in order, He... established the law of marriage, made it as a fortress for well-being and salvation...."[1] Bahá'u'lláh

There are these additional quotations that illuminate the foundation purposes of marriage and creating families:

"... Bahá'u'lláh has stated that the purpose of marriage is to promote unity...."[2]  On behalf of Shoghi Effendi

"... [T]he primary purpose of marriage is the procreation of children. A couple who are physically incapable of having children may, of course, marry, since the procreation of children is not the only purpose of marriage."[3]  On behalf of the Universal House of Justice

*Creating Well-Being for Couples and Families*

This short guidebook will show you new ways to enhance your couple and family well-being and share these concepts with others. Enjoy!

**Helpful Tips for Use:**

**Read:**

- Getting Started section
- Chapter 1 – Character
- And then go to whatever section you are interested in; using one section a day or one a week will keep you moving in a positive direction

**Order of the Sections:** There are many aspects of well-being included in this guide, but each section covers a standalone topic. You can choose a topic randomly, focus on a specific topic according to a current need, or go in order from the beginning (or ending!). It's completely up to you.

The initial part of the book focuses on physical well-being, somewhat like a warm-up activity before exercising, although there are many spiritual principles included. Relationship and family topics are then the focus. The book then includes topics with more spiritual focus. In an integrated life, all of these are woven together, and ideally, the spiritual focus becomes the larger context within which couples make decisions about physical, mental, emotional, and social well-being. As you consult together about well-being, you will engage in a process of calibrating all aspects of your life to create a coherent whole.

**Structure of Sections:** Each of the sections in this guide contains these components:

- **Reflections:** A quotation from another source and the author's comments on the topic

- **A Couple's Experience:** A short story that will provide ideas for applying the topic in your own lives
- **Well-Being Discussion:** Questions to help you understand and apply the topic
- **Learning Activities to Try:** Ideas of specific actions to move you forward
- **Conscious Focus:** A statement about your engagement with the topic of the section

**Growing Together:** Do your best to be open to this effort as a learning experience and avoid criticizing each other's actions. Your well-being is worth the time and focus! Not all suggestions will be a good fit for all couples or for all families. Please use wisdom and unified decision-making as you consider what to do and why.

Remember that making progress with enhancing well-being is a learning-in-action effort. It's not about perfection. You won't know the outcome until you:

- Try something
- Reflect on how it worked
- Discuss how it went and consult about what to do differently
- Repeat the same action or find a new one to take
- Then begin the cycle again

**Goal Setting:** There are suggested activities throughout this guide. Many of them include encouragement to do the activity for a week. Often you will choose to do it for longer, so it becomes a regular habit. It will be wise for you to have some type of system for setting and keeping track of your specific action goals and your progress toward them. There is an additional section at the end of the book about setting goals and achieving them over time. Remember, it will be best if your goals are:

- Clear
- Agreed-upon
- Attainable in a reasonable amount of time

## GETTING STARTED

**What is Well-Being?**

Science shows that involvement in social relationships benefits health. When both of you are demonstrating self-respect and happiness, you are more likely to be healthy. **Well-being** includes your physical health but goes beyond to include mental, emotional, social, and spiritual aspects. The Bahá'í teachings say this:

"... [M]an's supreme honor and real happiness lie in self-respect, in high resolves and noble purposes, in integrity and moral quality, in immaculacy of mind."[4] 'Abdu'l-Bahá

As a couple, the more you integrate and harmonize all aspects of health and create well-being, the happier you are likely to be. It works from the other direction too: The happier you are, the likelier you will both be healthy. With well-being, you feel more "in balance," and there is a "flow" of positive energy between you as a couple and between your activities.

When the two of you are healthy and happy together, you have more energy and time to parent well, see friends and family, and participate in your work and community service. You are present. You show up. You make a positive difference.

As you collaborate, accompany, and encourage each other, health and happiness increase. When you are united in creating well-being, you are healthier as individuals and in your relationship. Science has discovered this insight:

"Eating right and moving more—especially if we want to do these things on a regular basis and over a long span of time—are easier when we are inspired, cajoled, praised, and supported by the people who matter the most to us in our daily lives."[5] Thomas N. Bradbury, PhD, and Benjamin R. Karney, PhD

When you cooperate as a team, you are more likely to:

- Turn to each other to talk about your challenges
- Make and keep medical and dental appointments
- Eat healthier meals
- Reduce harmful habits
- Have stronger immune systems
- Seek help as needed
- Recover faster when you become ill

As equal partners, you look at the totality of your lives and choose the roles and responsibilities that are fair and respectful to both of you. You avoid the pitfalls of dominating each other, doing constant reminders, hiding behavior, or criticizing each other' actions. Instead, you look for ways to share your experiences, and you are more likely to encourage and help each other. You contribute to one another physically, mentally, emotionally, and spiritually.

**Being Intentional with Your Focus**

Creating couple well-being is an intentional choice and process. You:

- Consciously pause to assess what you are doing and why
- Envision the outcomes you want to achieve
- Make choices, decisions, and commitments as a couple about what is best for your individual and mutual health and happiness
- Choose the words and actions that create a good outcome

Your commitment to health and happiness is vital. Consider this wisdom:

"Until one is committed there is hesitancy, the chance to draw back, always ineffectiveness. Concerning all acts of initiative (and creation), there is one elementary truth, the ignorance of which kills countless ideas and splendid plans: that the moment one definitely commits oneself, then Providence moves too. All sorts of things occur to help one that would never otherwise have occurred. A whole stream of events issues from the decision, raising in one's favor all manner of unforeseen incidents and meetings and material assistance, which no man could have dreamt would have come his way."[6] W. H. Murray

Being intentional affects small and large choices in your life, such as for example:

- How often you pray
- How you manage household tasks
- How many hours a day you work and/or do service
- What major health and medical decisions you make

When you stop being conscious and intentional, you can ignore something that doesn't function well in your home, and you can neglect symptoms of illness. However, when you deny what is happening or stop paying attention, you are more likely to become ill, unhappy, or fight with each other. Doing a check on your reality and addressing what's happening in all areas of your lives, empowers you to be in action and reduces stress.

**Considering Your Priorities**

Couples have greater well-being when they are clear about their values, priorities, and purposes in life. These purposes are important drivers of your time and well-being priorities. Purposes could include striving for excellence with:

- Your relationship or marriage
- Parenting and family
- Spiritual activities
- Community service

- Profession
- Physical fitness

As you talk about what is important to both of you, consider in what ways you feel called to contribute to the lives of others, separately or together. When you know your purposes and priorities, being intentional empowers you to convert dreams into purposeful actions.

**Start Small and Grow Your Goals**

Translating your hopes and wishes into intentional action can seem daunting. It's often best to begin in small ways. Throughout this guide are action suggestions. Small ones are good to start with, such as:

- Pack healthier lunches
- Go for a walk one evening a week together
- Aim for 7-8 hours of sleep at least once a week
- Spend 10 minutes meditating together one morning a week

You can grow your goals over time and with practical and successful experiences. In this way, you will be intentionally creating your well-being as a couple and from you as a couple out to your family.

## 1 - CHARACTER

**Reflections:**

"The belief that we can rely on shortcuts to happiness, joy, rapture, comfort, and ecstasy, rather than be entitled to these feelings by the exercise of personal strengths and virtues, leads to legions of people who in the middle of great wealth are starving spiritually. Positive emotion alienated from the exercise of character leads to emptiness, to inauthenticity, to depression, and, as we age, to the gnawing realization that we are fidgeting until we die. The positive feeling that arises from the exercise of strengths and virtues, rather than from the shortcuts, is authentic."[7] Martin Seligman

"The foundation-stone of a life lived in the way of God is the pursuit of moral excellence and the acquisition of a character endowed with qualities that are well-pleasing in His sight."[8] Shoghi Effendi

"The power of God can entirely transmute our characters and make of us beings entirely unlike our previous selves. Through prayer and supplication, obedience to the divine laws Bahá'u'lláh has revealed, and ever-increasing service to His Faith, we can change ourselves."[9] On behalf of Shoghi Effendi

~~~

    This section will assist you with all the other sections. Character qualities or virtues are one of the best contributors to any happy person or relationship. When each of you demonstrates skill with character strengths; such as, caring, commitment, compassion, courage, courtesy, enthusiasm, flexibility, friendliness, generosity, helpfulness, integrity, respect, responsibility, thoughtfulness, trustworthiness, and truthfulness, you generate light in your hearts and souls as well as in your relationship. There is a deep feeling of well-being when these qualities show up in your words and actions.
    Of course, having strong character qualities is easier if you have focused on developing them from early childhood, which is why

raising children to have good characters is vital. If you begin to strengthen your character as an adult, the process is often more difficult, yet it's still essential. Transformation is always possible.

Sometimes change from outside of you can be a challenge and responding to it takes willingness and perseverance. Often, there is an internal prompt to change in response to difficulties or after you have made poor choices. Ongoing assessment, encouragement from people you trust and love, apologizing, practicing forgiveness, and making amends are all aspects of personal development. Sometimes you also benefit from remembering to lighten up and not take yourselves so seriously. Often the best way to handle mistakes is with a sense of humor.

Character qualities often balance each other when paired together, such as tactfulness along with truthfulness. Every quality is designed to create good results. However, you can cause harm if you apply them to excess or in the wrong time or place, or if you don't balance them with another quality. Another example is helpfulness, which is best paired with respect, as you then check if someone wants help and in what ways they are open to receiving it. Conscious application of the qualities is needed so the outcome is beneficial.

Pursuing and maintaining well-being also require applying character qualities. Possibilities might include creativity, gentleness, kindness, moderation, patience, perseverance, purposefulness, self-discipline, or wisdom.

**A Couple's Experience:**

*"What I love in our relationship is the regular practice of kind, courteous, and thoughtful actions of service to each other. These smooth the rough corners of life and assist us with appreciating each other. Fixing a meal, holding a door open, setting the table, getting the mail, providing a glass of water, checking the functioning of a vehicle, bringing a small gift, massaging a neck, providing reminders, and more all help our relationship and home flow more smoothly and peacefully."*

**Well-Being Discussion:**

- What are three character qualities that feel quite easy for each of us to practice? What are three that are more difficult?
- What assists us to make effective changes in our character? What can interfere?
- What qualities do we see as most beneficial to our lives? For us to practice with our children? For our children to have as strengths?

**Learning Activities to Try:**

- Choose two character qualities and practice them consistently for a week.
- Identify one character growth area for each of us, and do our best to turn it around to positive behavior for a week.
- Spend a day trying to find every possible way to think of the others in the home and respond with thoughtful acts of service.

**Conscious Focus:**

"We apply every character quality possible to our actions and relationship, including moderation."

## 2 – EXERCISE

**Reflections:**

"Athletics refresh the body, tranquilize and enlighten the mind, and develop moral character. As a concrete example let us take a student in his college activities. The student who does exercise is always fresh and vigorous, he seldom gets sick and tired. His jovial character, his good disposition and his interest in life are his chief characteristics.

"Moreover in exercising, the student gets animated, his blood is purified and consequently his mind becomes more apt to receive the ideas and thoughts found in his lessons. The health which he acquires will help him to work harder and he becomes more successful. A weak person seldom can endure the hardship of school-life, the trouble of memorizing and persevering in his daily lessons. Lastly when a student is busy with athletics during recess time his ideas do not deviate any more to the path of impurity, to think of such trivial things and the health and strength which he acquires will help him in overcoming such temptations. Generally a healthy person is endowed with a will stronger than that of a weak person."[10] Shoghi Effendi (before he was appointed the Guardian of the Bahá'í Faith)

"When you make realistic and gradual demands on the body, the body will develop. If equally progressive demands are made on the mind and emotions, they will develop as well."[11] Dan Millman

~~~

Regular physical exercise gradually conditions your bodies to be stronger and healthier. You then cope well with simple tasks like carrying groceries. You may also be able to engage in more complex activities like taking a hike on a hilly trail. Exercise requires self-discipline. It's often not easy to move when you are tired or get off the furniture when you are comfortable. You may benefit from examining and understanding the thoughts and emotions that interfere with choosing to exercise.

Exercising together can be an excellent way of helping each other move when you are inclined to resist. You may also discover games or sports you enjoy playing together. You may be a bit competitive in exercising, but don't take this to excess and get hurt. Exercising separately but with the goal of being strong and healthy for each other can also benefit your relationship.

Consider exercising your minds as well. This could include reading the same book, so you can have a lively discussion. You might access different sources of news and compare the perspectives you get from them. Think about what will stretch you out of your comfort zone intellectually and act on it.

Exercising self-discipline with your emotions can also benefit you. Controlling expressions of anger and increasing gratitude and acts of kindness can foster peace and unity between you. Regularly practicing and strengthening your ability to express love and compassion can contribute to a great relationship.

When you think of spiritual exercise, it might include reading spiritual materials, meditation, or being consistent with saying certain prayers. There will be more on this topic later in the guide.

**A Couple's Experience:**

*"When we began dating, we were both exercising regularly. One of us swam a lot, and the other did strengthening at the gym and rode a bike. We tried exercising together, but it just didn't seem to work well. Our bodies needed different activities, and our schedules didn't mesh well for exercising. We found after marriage that we both enjoy going on walks together, and this is good exercise and couple time. However, we generally still do serious exercise separately.*

*"We made a promise to each other to do our best to accomplish some form of exercise daily and let the other know about it. We don't hit this goal 100%, but the promise keeps us in action. We congratulate each other on our achievements. We are committed to being active throughout our lives."*

**Well-Being Discussion:**

- What are our patterns and choices with stretching and exercise? What parts of our bodies could benefit from doing less? Doing more?
- What are our realistic goals for physical improvement? Mental improvement? Emotional improvement? Spiritual improvement?
- What types of activities are tiring and leave us feeling poorly? Which are invigorating and increase feelings of well-being?

**Learning Activities to Try:**

- Choose one physical fitness or sports activity to do two-three times this week together.
- Learn about and encourage each other's exercise goals; praise achievements.
- Read and discuss an article or book about physical or mental fitness.

**Conscious Focus:**

"We increase our energy and accomplishments when we keep our bodies strong."

## 3 - NUTRITION

**Reflections:**

"When highly skilled physicians shall fully examine this matter, thoroughly and perseveringly, it will be clearly seen that the incursion of disease is due to a disturbance in the relative amounts of the body's component substances, and that treatment consisteth in adjusting these relative amounts, and that this can be apprehended and made possible by means of foods.

"It is certain that in this wonderful new age the development of medical science will lead to the doctors' healing their patients with foods. For the sense of sight, the sense of hearing, of taste, of smell, of touch—all these are discriminative faculties, their purpose being to separate the beneficial from whatever causeth harm."[12] 'Abdu'l-Bahá

"Many of us have swallowed the idea that when it comes to food, faster is better. We are in a hurry, and we want meals to match. But many people are waking up to the drawbacks of the gobble-gulp-and-go ethos. On the farm, in the kitchen and at the table, they are slowing down."[13] Carl Honoré

~~~

Food nourishes your bodies. When you maintain excellent nutrition, your bodies function better, your thinking is clearer and more effective, and your emotions are more likely to stay stable or rebalance easily. If you choose simple, high-quality food, well-being is likelier to occur. Your nutrition choices can prevent illness. If you help each other grow, buy, cook, and eat good food, meals become pleasurable occasions.

Science is still uncovering knowledge about food and how it behaves in our bodies and influences health or causes illness. Every person's body is unique, and foods and supplements behave differently for each person.

However, there are general principles that will usually guide you in a beneficial direction:

- Fresh and simple foods
- Minimally processed and affected by chemicals
- Variety of colors and flavors
- Fruits, vegetables, proteins, and grains in balance
- Clean water purifies and hydrates your bodies, which are composed of a large amount of water

**A Couple's Experience:**

"We began with one of us mostly vegetarian and the other eating meat regularly. We decided to experiment with meeting in the middle and eating more of each other's choices, while also listening to the needs of our individual bodies. Over time, we discovered intolerance issues with some grains, and that caused us to make further adjustments.

"We have two sons now, and they have their own needs and desires for us to manage. However, unity is always important to us, so we choose to eat as a family and strive to eat as close to the same thing as possible. It's just too difficult to prepare separate meals. Often, we eat slightly different meals, but we do it together."

**Well-Being Discussion:**

- How do foods and nutritional supplements seem to affect our bodies? Moods? Energy levels? What changes do we want to make?
- What are our views about home cooking from fresh ingredients rather than eating out at restaurants or buying pre-prepared foods? How can we increase the number of home-cooked meals we consume as a couple? As a family?
- How are meals different when we eat on the run or separately compared to when we sit down together as a couple or family (without the TV on and accessing electronic devices)? How

does it feel when we invite friends to our home and share food with them?

**Learning Activities to Try:**

- Keep food diaries for a few days or a week, noting what we ate and how we felt as a result. What foods make us feel poorly or positively, such as heavy, energized, achy, tired, light, heavy, bloated, or satisfied?
- Research two foods that we eat regularly to understand what they are composed of and their potential benefits.
- Plan a simple, nutritious meal and invite another couple or family to eat with us.

**Conscious Focus:**

"We value the strength and vitality that comes from excellent nutrition."

## 4 - RELAXATION

**Reflections:**

"...[Y]ou should not neglect your health, but consider it the means which enables you to serve. It—the body—is like a horse which carries the personality and spirit, and as such should be well cared for so it can do its work! You should certainly safeguard your nerves, and force yourself to take time, and not only for prayer and meditation, but for real rest and relaxation. We don't have to pray and meditate for hours in order to be spiritual."[14]  On behalf of Shoghi Effendi

"The most relaxing recreating forces are a healthy religion, sleep, music, and laughter. Have faith in God—learn to sleep well—love good music—see the funny side of life—and health and happiness will be yours."[15] Dale Carnegie

~~~

When excessive tension builds up in your bodies, minds, hearts, and souls, it causes vulnerability to illness. Relaxation of your nerves strengthens your immune systems and allows you to regenerate energy. With relaxation, the chatter or noise in your minds calms down, and your thoughts clarify. It's easier to feel open to spiritual influences. It's easier to feel loving.

Everyone's environment and life are different. What is relaxing for one person can produce tension in another. This can be true for couples as well and will also likely vary among your children. The key is observing and learning what does relax you and including it in balance in your life together. Ideally, you will discover at least one activity that relaxes each of you. Hopefully, you will find more than one!

Relaxation in balance aids your effectiveness with your work and service choices. Sometimes people who are dedicating their lives to contribute to others forget to take care of themselves. It can be easy to be in the mindset of always sacrificing oneself. However, this approach can cause physical, mental, emotional, and spiritual burnout, not something that serves others for the long-term.

**A Couple's Experience:**

*"We enjoy our work and service most of the time, but this can lead us to being active all of the time. We have deliberately set up our home environment to include places where relaxation happens naturally. There are comfortable chairs with a lovely view. There are places to walk with trees and flowers. What supports our relaxation are: time in meditation, photography, reading a novel, regular hugs, some movies, laughing, physical intimacy, and a comfortable bed mattress and pillows."*

**Well-Being Discussion:**

- What facilitates us relaxing separately? Together? How does harmony in our relationship affect our ability to relax? When we are relaxed, how does that affect our children?
- When does a need to "be in control" or "be responsible" interfere with our ability to relax?
- What benefit does relaxation bring to our bodies, minds, hearts, and souls?

**Learning Activities to Try:**

- Hold each other or snuggle for two-five minutes or until we both feel our muscles relax.
- Try these activities and assess what is (or is not!) relaxing or uplifting: watch a comedy show or movie, listen to different types of music, do yoga or a similar practice, play a game, do a craft, cook together, sit in the sunshine, and read a book aloud to each other.
- Fix tea, coffee, or some other drink and share positive experiences from the day while drinking, ensuring that our children are trained to respect this couple time except in

emergencies. Alternatively, each person can share their day over a family meal.

**Conscious Focus:**

"We relax ourselves—mentally, emotionally, physically, and spiritually—at appropriate times—to regenerate and empower us to operate at peak efficiency throughout life."

## 5 - SLEEP

**Reflections:**

"... [T]here are very few people who can get along without eight hours sleep. If you are not one of those, you should protect your health by sleeping enough. The Guardian [Shoghi Effendi]...finds that it impairs his working capacity if he does not try and get a minimum of seven or eight hours."[16]  On behalf of Shoghi Effendi

"How close you feel to your partner, how secure you feel in the relationship, and how many positive emotions you readily attribute to your relationship are all closely tied to sleep quality. Evidence shows, for example, that spouses with fewer sleep problems also tend to be happier. It could be that relationship woes make for poorer quality sleep, or that a bad night's sleep affects one's relationship—but the likely case is one of bi-directional influence. In other words, chances are that changing one's sleep habits might improve relationship quality."[17]  Theresa E. DiDonato, PhD

~~~

Good quality sleep allows your brains to sort out and file information. It allows your bodies to relax and regenerate their stores of energy. Hormones have the chance to rebalance. Lack of adequate sleep contributes to accidents, diseases, and poor judgment.

Getting enough rest is especially challenging for parents of babies and young children. Parents often must take turns responding during the night to protect each other's health. Parents can also look for ways to grab daytime naps. Naps and nighttime rest are vital for restoring well-being and energy. Getting enough sleep contributes to the physical, mental, emotional, and spiritual aspects of your lives.

Sleeping positions, touching or not touching, snoring or other noises, twitching, physical impairment, illness, disturbing dreams, need for different temperatures, and more can make sharing bed space a challenge. It can also be a challenge when a couple is on different sleep schedules due to work or biological clocks. You may have to try very hard and be creative with solutions to stay sleeping together. You may also discover it builds connection at times to "visit" each other in bed for couple cuddling before needing to be in separate places. If one of you must get up before the other, having activities or a light meal while waiting for the other to rise can contribute to keeping your relationship peaceful.

Some couples and other family members benefit from a period of unwinding before bed, without TV, phones, computers, and other devices. Light can also be an issue, and you can experiment with darker curtains, eye masks, and dimmable overhead lights. Making sure these physical needs are addressed can lead to healthier sleep patterns.

**A Couple's Experience:**

*"Our children are now old enough to sleep through the night, but we find that we still struggle to make sleep a priority. When the kids are in bed, we finally have a chance to have a little time to ourselves, and to spend time together as a couple. We frequently stay up too late because we don't want this precious time to be over! But, that's a set-up for exhaustion the next day, which translates to low productivity and short tempers.*

*"We are trying to find the middle road, in which we make sleep the top priority while not totally sacrificing our free time. Discussing it together and making the commitment to get more sleep is helping a great deal. Also, we've found that computers, social media, and electronics suck up time in the evening, and we are getting better at turning them off. We're trying to be more mindful about our activities so that we can really maximize our couple time."*

**Well-Being Discussion:**

- How do we feel when we have had enough sleep? How does it affect our relationships and functioning?

- When do we use naps and rest breaks to compensate for lack of sleep?
- What helps us feel sleepier? Sleep more soundly?

**Learning Activities to Try:**

- Pick a night of the week or time period each evening before bed that we agree will be free of electronic devices or try some other new evening routine.
- For a week, record how many hours of sleep we get, the quality of the sleep, and how we feel in the morning. Assess what to change and then try the changed pattern for a week.
- Make changes in our sleeping environment, such as adding padding to make our mattress softer or putting a board under the mattress to make it more firm, change types of pillows, add black-out curtains, play white noise, use earplugs, or sleep with a cooler temperature with air conditioning, a fan on, or windows open.

**Conscious Focus:**

"We allow our bodies to deeply rest and recover each day."

# 6 - ILLNESS

**Reflections:**

"There are two ways of healing sickness, material means and spiritual means. The first is by the treatment of physicians; the second consisteth in prayers offered by the spiritual ones to God and in turning to Him. Both means should be used and practiced.
"Illnesses which occur by reason of physical causes should be treated by doctors with medical remedies; those which are due to spiritual causes disappear through spiritual means. Thus an illness caused by affliction, fear, nervous impressions, will be healed more effectively by spiritual rather than by physical treatment."[18] 'Abdu'l-Bahá

Excerpt from section "How to Stay Well (or Get Better...)":
"5. Love yourself, and love everyone else. Make loving the purpose and primary expression in your life.
"6. Create fun, loving, honest relationships, allowing for the expression and fulfillment of needs for intimacy and security...."[19] Bernie S. Siegel, MD

~~~

There is a significant amount of science showing the health benefits of marriage, including living longer. Couple behavior in general though is part of protecting your health and well-being. You care about each other, so you care about each other's health. You encourage each other to visit the dentist and doctor for checkups and treatment. You keep your bodies clean and healthy, so you don't negatively affect each other. You do spiritual activities together such as prayer. All of these types of actions are positive examples for children and encourage them to be healthy as well.

Couples are more likely to address physical wellness issues rather than ignoring them. You are more likely to eat healthier meals together. Loving touch happens more often. Sex or other types of intimacy are more frequent. You listen to each other's troubles and help each other through them. Overall, you know there is someone watching out for your well-being.

When illness, accidents, or injuries happen, being a couple means you have someone to advocate on your behalf with healthcare professionals. You encourage or participate in treatments and lift each other's spirits. Together you learn about what is happening and how to address it in effective and healing ways. You persevere together through the treatment and response period. You are more likely to recover and recover well with mutual support.

**A Couple's Experience:**

*"We don't get sick very often, but when we do, there is usually something emotional that has lowered our immune systems. It could be stress related to criticism from someone at work, missing an important deadline, or an upset family member. It's often the same if we have a minor injury, like a sprained ankle—fatigue or emotional distraction are often factors that contributed to the accident.*

*"We have learned that we need to talk together about what is affecting our emotions and how they are affecting what is happening physically. Sometimes we must enlist healthcare practitioners to help us understand what is happening too. When we have these insights, using supplements, foods, and medical treatments can work better to heal the physical side of the illness or injury. We notice that collaborating together on healing makes it much easier to be consistent with the treatments until well-being returns."*

**Well-Being Discussion:**

- What do we do to prevent or minimize physical illnesses?
- How do we handle stress or emotional upsets that could lead to physical illnesses or injuries?
- What ways do we help each other through illnesses or injuries? Where do we want to improve our responses?

**Learning Activities to Try:**

- Identify and take three supplements that can maintain well-being and that won't interfere with any medications we are taking.
- Stock our home with what would help us effectively prevent or respond to common cold or flu symptoms.
- Develop a list of two to three questions to ask when something happens to identify if there is an emotional cause to consider as a factor in an illness or injury.

**Conscious Focus:**

"We focus on preventing illness and injury and then restoring wellness as soon as something occurs."

## 7 - TIME

**Reflections:**

"Relationships grow from connection, not from performance or management. To connect you must slow down, attend, disclose yourself, and nurture. ... Driving yourself with an excessive need for efficiency does not lead to more time spent relaxing; it simply leads to more time spent stewing over whether you could have gotten through yet another moment of your life more quickly. ... In both relationships and work, the best antidote to burnout is engaging in pleasure and playfulness. ... Romance, nurturing, communication, and intimacy require energy. You can't exhaust yourself and remain an effective partner or lover."[20]
Wayne M. Sotile, PhD, and Mary O. Sotile, MA

"... [E]xercise moderation in all things. Whatsoever passeth beyond the limits of moderation will cease to exert a beneficial influence."[21]
Bahá'u'lláh

"... [T]he unity of your family should take priority over any other consideration. Bahá'u'lláh came to bring unity to the world, and a fundamental unity is that of the family. ...[S]ervice ... should not produce neglect of the family. It is important for you to arrange your time so that your family life is harmonious and your household receives the attention it requires."[22]  On behalf of the Universal House of Justice

~~~

Couples come in every shape, size, color, personality, and range of interests possible. One couple fosters their relationship by watching TV together most nights. Another couple is deeply involved in community activities many days a week. Yet another focuses on their children's activities. Achieving a sense of balance or coherence across all aspects of life is often very difficult, but vital. Well-being can suffer otherwise.

Setting priorities for your usage of time links back to the Getting Started section of this guide that mentioned "being intentional". What you consciously choose to do with your time is most effective when it connects with your stated purposes in life and what you value. Maintaining your couple well-being is a very important priority that helps you fulfill your purposes. As you keep your relationship healthy, it contributes an important example to others. Your words and actions encourage well-being in your friends and family.

Individuals and couples living in a fast-paced world may get stuck in thinking that they must do everything and be everything for everyone. When you understand your purposes, values, and priorities, you increase your ability to politely say "no" to some choices. When you understand the importance of well-being, you can also begin to see where you need to say "yes" to choices that support it.

**A Couple's Experience:**

*"We were asked to do 'one more thing' to benefit our community, and we knew if we said 'yes', it would be too much. We both spent time in reflection, writing down all we were doing, who we were serving, who requested us to do these actions, and our motivations for being involved. We talked about who else could do part of our work and service commitments.*

*"We assessed the effect on our marriage and family of every item, and we looked at the overall quality and quantity of what we were doing. This detailed process helped us feel more in control of our time and choices. We were able to say 'no' to some things, 'yes' to others, and modify yet others. What a relief!"*

**Well-Being Discussion:**

- In what ways do our work and community service activities benefit each other and others?

- What happens to our relationship when we feel pulled many directions and stop having time to connect with each other and our family?
- Are we spending time on what we consider our highest priorities? Are there invisible time-suckers such as watching media and participating in social media? Are there hobbies or activities we are overly dependent on that need to be addressed?

**Learning Activities to Try:**

- Track our major time choices for a week (or month) and then discuss what changes to make.
- Think about any unfulfilled dreams and goals we each have and discuss how to fulfill them.
- Spend time doing something together we find attractive and that we don't usually do.

**Conscious Focus:**

"We spend the time needed to safeguard the well-being of our relationship and family."

## 8 - FRIENDSHIP

**Reflections:**

"The Lord, peerless is He, hath made woman and man to abide with each other in the closest companionship, and to be even as a single soul. They are two helpmates, two intimate friends, who should be concerned about the welfare of each other."[23] 'Abdu'l-Bahá

"… [H]appy marriages are based on a deep friendship. By this I mean a mutual respect for and enjoyment of each other's company. These couples tend to know each other intimately—they are well versed in each other's likes, dislikes, personality quirks, hopes, and dreams. They have an abiding regard for each other and express this fondness not just in the big ways but through small gestures day in and day out. … Friendship fuels the flames of romance because it offers the best protection against feeling adversarial toward your spouse. … In the strongest marriages, husband and wife share a deep sense of meaning. They don't just "get along"—they also support each other's hopes and aspirations and build a sense of purpose into their lives together."[24] John M. Gottman, PhD, and Nan Silver

~~~

Friendship is a factor in any relationship that contributes to it lasting. In an intimate relationship, friendship is part of being companions and helpmates who care about each other's well-being. You understand and appreciate each other and enjoy each other's company. You find it easy to laugh together. You are each other's primary confidant, and you keep what each other says as private. You guard each other from the negative words and actions of others. Your affection for each other shows in small and large actions every day and provides a strong sense of security and well-being for your children.

With a close friendship between you, it's possible to relax and share what is on your minds and in your hearts. You know what you share will be respected and appreciated. When you share thoughts and make mutual decisions about life, beliefs, children, jobs, community service, or other matters of importance, you come to understand one another's values and purposes in life. You can share your perspectives and strengthen your unity. You build a life history together.

There are vital character qualities that are part of being best friends and maintaining your friendship, such as:

- Loyalty
- Honesty
- Respect
- Trust

When you treat each other as close friends, your confidence in your relationship grows. You want to spend time with one another. You encourage and help one another through difficulties, times of personal growth, and toward achieving goals. You sincerely celebrate with each other's achievements and triumphs.

**A Couple's Experience:**

*"When one of us was chosen to lead a major project at work, the first thought was to share the news with the other and celebrate together. When one of our parents became critically ill, the other was there with a hug and helping to arrange travel. We cuddle on the couch with tea or fruit smoothies and share about our days.*

*"We look for ways to uplift each other during difficult times with special foods, flowers, text messages with quotations, and more. We enjoy traveling new places together. We laugh (kindly) about personality quirks in ourselves and family members. We speak lovingly and respectfully to each other. We see each other's friendship as a blessing and a gift."*

**Well-Being Discussion:**

- What signs in our relationship show that we are friends?

- What aspects of friendship do we want to strengthen? How will this benefit us and our children?
- How does having other individual and couple friends help us value friendship in our couple relationship? Would it benefit us to have more friends? Spend time more often with friends? Invite friends to visit us?

**Learning Activities to Try:**

- Share about something that happened recently in our lives together or separately and express our thoughts and feelings about it.
- Offer to do something for the other that they dislike doing.
- Identify another couple whose friendship we admire and invite them to spend time with us talking about friendship.

**Conscious Focus:**

"We enjoy each other's company as intimate friends."

## 9 - DATES

**Reflections:**

"Great dates are more than going to see a movie and tuning out the world for a while. Great dates involve communicating with one another, reviving the spark that initially ignited your fire, and developing mutual interests and goals that are not focused on your careers or your children. Great dates can revitalize your relationship."[25] Claudia Arp and David Arp

"... [M]arriage can be a source of well-being, conveying a sense of security and spiritual happiness. However, it is not something that just happens. For marriage to become a haven of contentment it requires the cooperation of the marriage partners themselves, and the assistance of their families...."[26] On behalf of the Universal House of Justice

~~~

Spending pleasant relaxing social time with each other can soften how you see each other and increases your sense of well-being. It's easier to laugh, smile, and be friends. What you choose to do as date-type activities can vary widely. However, it's wise to consider how the activity could contribute to your relationship or potentially harm it. Then you can consciously choose what is best.

Social times are not opportunities to coordinate the administrative details of your lives. They are not the time to raise topics that will sabotage the mood and insert disunity. It's a time to catch up with each other's lives and enjoy sharing thoughts and dreams.

Money, childcare helpers such as family or friends you trust, and available time all affect your choices. However, dates don't have to be about spending money or even being out of the house. They can be special times set up to be in a "bubble" where the two of you are only what matters at that moment.

Part of your social life can be offering hospitality, if this is something you both enjoy, and it enhances your lives and those of your guests. Inviting people to your home can prompt you to clean and organize. Hospitality gives you the opportunity to try out new foods and activities. It can be like having a date in your own home.

Socializing assists you with building friendships with others. Building good friendships with others creates a support system that you can count on when an aspect of your lives is disrupted. As you greet and serve people together as a couple, it links you more tightly together.

**A Couple's Experience:**

*"We found that every date was just going to dinner at the same places, and that was getting boring. Now we do Alphabet Dates each week, where we take turns and create a date that begins with a specific letter. It's fun and a surprise for the other person. Last week I had the letter "B" and did Breakfast for dinner, a Bed made of Blankets on the Beach, along with Books to read. It's fun to spend the week thinking about what to come up with for the letter and have that to look forward to."*

**Well-Being Discussion:**

- What is our pattern of leisure/social time together? What do we want to change so that time alone together is sometimes a priority?
- What will contribute to us enjoying social activities together?
- What do we see as the purposes and benefits of offering hospitality? What challenges might we have to overcome to host people in our home?

**Learning Activities to Try:**

- Watch a movie together while touching and sharing refreshments.

- Participate in an activity that is a special interest for one or both of us.
- Find someone trustworthy to be with our children and go out on a fun or relaxing date.

**Conscious Focus:**

"We enjoy participating in social times that refresh and enliven our relationship."

## 10 - CLEANLINESS

**Reflections:**

"Even in the physical realm, cleanliness will conduce to spirituality…. And although bodily cleanliness is a physical thing, it hath, nevertheless, a powerful influence on the life of the spirit. It is even as a voice wondrously sweet, or a melody played: although sounds are but vibrations in the air which affect the ear's auditory nerve, and these vibrations are but chance phenomena carried along through the air, even so, see how they move the heart. A wondrous melody is wings for the spirit, and maketh the soul to tremble for joy. The purport is that physical cleanliness doth also exert its effect upon the human soul."[27] 'Abdu'l-Bahá

"Cleanliness means washing often, keeping your body clean, and wearing clean clothes. … Cleanliness can be in your mind as well as your body. A clean mind means that you keep your thoughts on things which are good for you. You can 'clean up your act' by deciding to change when you have done something you aren't proud of or when you have made a mistake. It is 'wiping the slate clean' and starting over when you want to improve yourself. 'Staying clean' also means keeping your body free of harmful drugs."[28] Linda Kavelin Popov

~~~

Water is an amazing gift in achieving cleanliness. It can also soothe, warm, cool, heal, and relax your bodies. When you are clean, you feel uplifted and balanced, and your spirits feel refreshed and alive. Being clean makes touching each other a more positive experience, including being sexually intimate.

Cleanliness is also about keeping your environment fresh and orderly. Assess how you each feel when things are dirty or messy and then try the opposite. Perhaps your preferences about clutter fall in the middle somewhere. It's also good to assess how attractive your environment is to both of you. This can include furniture, decorations, or location. You may have accumulated items that no longer have an emotional or functional significance, and cleaning them out of the environment is wise. Teaching your children to participate in cleaning, organizing, and de-cluttering will be important skill-building for them in life.

Cleanliness is sometimes linked with the quality of purity, which can also apply to your thoughts, activities, and choices. A pure mind is protected from strong and negative emotions like anger, hatred, or jealousy. Inputs like pornography or violence can disturb your purity, your sense of inner cleanliness. Avoiding them helps keep your mind, heart, and body clean. Someone with a pure character is more likely to behave with kindness, courtesy, and compassion. Seeking purity of spirit or soul can lead to finding solace, help, and peace through prayer and meditation.

**A Couple's Experience:**

*"It has become couple time for us to be in the bathroom together near bedtime. We brush our teeth, carry on a conversation, remind each other of tasks to do in the morning, and clean our bodies. When we lived on our own, we showered at different times of the day. When we married and began living together, we discovered we loved the couple connection and mutual relaxation involved in showering together before bed in the evenings. Sometimes we also enjoy filling our tub with hot water and salts of some type and soaking to relax our muscles as well as get clean."*

**Well-Being Discussion:**

- How do we feel when we have immersed in water and become clean?
- How do we feel when our environment is clean? Orderly? Attractive?
- What thoughts and emotions are happening regularly that we feel need "cleansing"? How can we accomplish this?

**Learning Activities to Try:**

- Choose an area of our home we want to be cleaner and more orderly and work together to accomplish it.
- Identify someone that we have been backbiting about and criticizing and discover positive words to say about the person's positive qualities instead.
- Watch three different types of movies and assess how clean our minds and spirits feel afterward.

**Conscious Focus:**

"We love to have clean bodies, minds, hearts, and souls."

## 11 - SEX

**Reflections:**

"Pleasure, variety, passion, and fun are not the goals of sex, but by-products of a mature, caring, God-honoring love life. The true goal of sex is a sacred, mysterious oneness. Fulfilling sex can only be an outgrowth of the genuine freedom that comes as another gift from a loving God."[29] Tim Alan Gardner

"While recognizing the Divine origin and force of the sex impulse in man, religion teaches that it must be controlled, and Bahá'u'lláh's Law confines its expression to the marriage relationship."[30] On behalf of the Universal House of Justice

"... [S]ecure bonding and fully satisfying sexuality go hand in hand; they cue off and enhance each other. Emotional connection creates great sex, and great sex creates deeper emotional connection. When partners are emotionally accessible, responsive, and engaged, sex becomes intimate play, a safe adventure. Secure partners feel free and confident to surrender to sensation in each other's arms, explore and fulfill their sexual needs, and share their deepest joys, longings, and vulnerabilities. Then, lovemaking is truly making love."[31] Sue Johnson

~~~

Sexual experiences can create a strong experience of oneness between you as a couple that can contribute to all aspects of your relationship. The intimacy that you build through sharing other harmonious experiences also enhances the oneness you experience in bed. Intimacy in lovemaking is not just a physical connection between you as partners; it is also a joining of your hearts and souls.

Applying your sexual energy and expressions in positive, relationship-building ways, will enhance your overall well-being. This includes treating each other with deep love, respect, and faithfulness. Sexual intimacy is designed to build connection and unity between you in a healthy way. Positive sexual energy is disrupted in couples when there is regular disunity, or there are actions such as infidelity, pornography, addiction, abusive experiences, and more. Addressing these generally requires professional and spiritual counseling as well as other supportive resources or groups.

It's important for well-being that you place sex in a balanced perspective as a positive part of a full and satisfying life together, not as the centerpiece. This can be difficult if either of you feels your needs are not being met. Open communication, expressing what you need and want and are willing to do or not do, and cooperating to find solutions will assist sex to be an important but not a dominant part of your relationship. Often learning about your bodies and about how to have positive sexual experiences can also make a vital difference.

**A Couple's Experience:**

*"The experience of touching each other deeply fulfills our need for love and caring. Often, we see a blend between our physical and spiritual feelings towards each other. We have no sense of sex as 'unclean" or 'bad' but rather view it as a way to joyfully connect. As our bodies change throughout life, we notice a need for flexibility, humor, cooperation, and understanding. We also see how important it is to stay as physically fit as possible."*

**Well-Being Discussion:**

- What would show that we are making our sexual time together an important priority?
- What new words and actions could we try to see if they enhance our intimate experience?
- How can we increase our sense of feeling united through sexual intimacy?

**Learning Activities to Try:**

- Greet each other with physical affection after being apart.
- Engage in sex spontaneously. As needed instead, agree on a time to be intimate when there will be few distractions (especially children), and fully engage in the experience.
- Pray with each other to have a unifying sexual experience.

**Conscious Focus:**

"We appreciate being in harmony with each other through physical and sexual touch."


**Note:** Couples who are experiencing serious disruptions in their sex life for any reason, such as significant differences in libido, infidelity, illness, or use of pornography, are wise to consult educational resources and professionals.

## 12 - PARENTING

**Reflections:**

"Thus the husband and wife are brought into affinity, are united and harmonized, even as though they were one person. Through their mutual union, companionship and love great results are produced in the world, both material and spiritual. The spiritual result is the appearance of divine bounties. The material result is the children who are born in the cradle of love of God, who are nurtured by the breast of the knowledge of God, and who are brought up in the bosom of the gift of God, and who are fostered in the lap of the training of God."[32] 'Abdu'l-Bahá

"Adjustments [to having a child] ...are natural and inevitable. But there is a difference between adjusting your marriage to meet your children's needs and losing your marriage to parenthood. ... Children are natural and eager consumers of whatever time, attention, and goods and services that parents will provide. It's the job of parents to discern how much is enough, how much is too much, and to enforce the difference. ... The greater danger for most of us is to lose our marriage to the demands of parenthood rather than losing our kids to the demands of our marriage (although this happens sometimes in stepfamilies). In a two-parent family, we either fight to create and keep a marriage-centered family, in which the couple relationship is the stable fulcrum of the family and the couple together care for their children, or we become a child-centered family in which the marriage goes on the shelf."[33] William J. Doherty, PhD

~~~

One of the greatest joys and one of the greatest challenges for a couple is becoming and being parents. It can be very easy to lose track of the priority of your couple relationship when becoming a family. It's wise to remember that the strength and closeness between the two of you is a significant contributor to the security and well-being of your children. It's also vital for your own well-being. Then after you go through all the challenges of raising children, it will be a challenge when the children leave, and you become a couple again!

There is an abundance of parenting advice available. You can learn from experts and other parents, and this is wise. However, you must determine for yourselves what type of parents you want to be and how to function as a family. Just as every child is different, so is every parent and family. Education, discipline, and physical care all vary by person. You will clarify your family values, make the time choices that work well for you, and respect the needs and rights of each family member. You will have to determine together how you will keep your own relationship a high priority in the mix.

**A Couple's Experience:**

*"In the weeks after our daughter was born, we felt like we were moving in a fog of exhaustion. Other than an occasional hug, we barely felt like a couple. Then one morning after a few hours of sleep, we realized we missed each other! We consulted with my mother who lived nearby. She agreed to come over after the baby was asleep and be there for an hour.*

*"We only went to a local restaurant for dessert, but that was enough to remind us that we had non-baby things to talk about and a friendship and couple relationship to maintain. We committed to continue going out on dates every few weeks, and we have kept it up through several years of parenting and the arrival of a second child. It was one of the best decisions we ever made."*

**Well-Being Discussion:**

- What learning could we access to increasingly strengthen our ability to be excellent parents?
- What can help us to have adult conversations that do not revolve around the children? How are we doing with maintaining adult relationships with friends? Are there changes we want to make?

- What activities do we most enjoy doing with our children as a family?

**Learning Activities to Try:**

- Depending on their ages, initiate or participate in Bahá'í-based children's classes or arrange for our children to participant in a junior youth spiritual empowerment group or study circles in our area.
- Find other parents rearing children similar in age with our children and do an activity together.
- Participate in a spiritual activity as a family.

**Conscious Focus:**

"We maintain our relationship as a high priority while also building a unified and healthy family."

## 13 - FAMILY

**Reflections:**

"... [T]he family, being a human unit, must be educated according to the rules of sanctity. All the virtues must be taught the family. The integrity of the family bond must be constantly considered, and the rights of the individual members must not be transgressed. The rights of the son, the father, the mother—none of them must be transgressed, none of them must be arbitrary. Just as the son has certain obligations to his father, the father, likewise, has certain obligations to his son. The mother, the sister and other members of the household have their certain prerogatives. The injury of one shall be considered the injury of all; the comfort of each, the comfort of all; the honor of one, the honor of all."[34]  'Abdu'l-Bahá

"Because keeping commitments has such an impact on trust—and because trust is so vital to a thriving family culture—it's wise to keep in mind that commitments to family members are often the most important commitments of all. Also...making and keeping commitments to yourself is the key to success in making and keeping commitments to others. That's where it all starts, and that's what gives you the power and the confidence—the Self Trust—that enables you to build trust with others."[35] Stephen M. R. Covey

~~~

Creating family unity is a unique challenge for all parents. Part of what keeps families intact is respect for each person involved. Family loyalty, where you all feel like you are on each other's side, can be part of what keeps unity in place. Family meetings, where each person has a voice, can be a way to build and maintain unity. Other mutual activities can build excellent experiences that create precious memories.

It's highly likely that there are more involved in your lives besides just the two of you and any children or stepchildren you have. Maybe there are parents or grandparents. There could be aunts, uncles, or cousins. Maybe there are former relatives that still feel like family. Maybe there are close friends that you treat like family. You each have histories with this complex mix of people, and maybe some old hurts that have never quite healed.

Family relationships can be an interesting puzzle to maintain. Who you choose to spend time with or interact with can contribute to your healthy relationship as a couple and the well-being of your children. Alternatively, some family members could regularly trigger irritation and disunity.

As you look over the array of people who have been in your lives and those who are still around, take the time to understand what relationships are healthy. Where they are unhealthy, can you heal the issues? Where is it emotionally or physically unsafe and so it's wise to set a boundary and lovingly detach from being around another person? Which relationships contribute happiness and enrichment to your lives? Which relationships do you want to strengthen?

You cannot choose all your family members, but you can choose your level of involvement with them. Assess and choose as best as you can what contributes to your couple and family well-being.

**A Couple's Experience:**

*"With everyone busy with their own lives and responsibilities, we have found it challenging to bring scattered family members together. It's often the best approach to meet over a meal, whether at our home, one of their homes, or at a restaurant. Eating together relaxes and re-connects us as we share stories about what is happening in our lives. Inevitably, stories from the past arise as well, usually with laughter."*

**Well-Being Discussion:**

- How do we maintain unified relationships amongst ourselves who live in the same home? With our extended family that live elsewhere?
- What extended family members do we really enjoy spending time with? Which ones seem to be troublesome? Why? Can something be addressed to improve the situation?
- How are extended family relationships affecting our unity as a couple? As a family?

**Learning Activities to Try:**

- Schedule special time as a couple (or include children), to visit with key family members, including perhaps reaching out to an estranged family member and re-establishing a healthier connection.
- Do an art activity, such as drawing a family tree, or participate in a community service project with extended family members.
- Begin a practice of having regular family meetings, choosing ahead which roles people will fill (chair, note-taker), identifying the topic(s) to cover, and gathering the facts needed for an effective consultation.

**Conscious Focus:**

"We appreciate building relationships with our extended family."

## 14 - WORK

**Reflections:**

"It is enjoined upon every one of you to engage in some form of occupation.... Waste not your time in idleness and sloth. Occupy yourselves with that which profiteth yourselves and others. ... When anyone occupieth himself in a craft or trade, such occupation itself is regarded in the estimation of God as an act of worship; and this is naught but a token of His infinite and all-pervasive bounty."[36] Bahá'u'lláh

"This marvelous capacity we have to do, to produce, is at once the spring of our health and, to a great extent, our happiness in life. Nothing can convey so solid a feeling of satisfaction in this world as something we have accomplished. A job well done, be it making a pie or writing a book or building a bridge, can produce a degree of contentment, a sense of buoyancy and fulfillment, that practically nothing else can. ... Because work is necessary for us, it sets the very essence of our being in circulation, and just as the blood performs so many services in our body essential to health, such as carrying away impurities, re-oxygenizing itself in the lungs, bringing food to the tissues, so work seems to give tone to our whole machine, exhilarates us, and calls forth a new flow of energy."[37] Rúhíyyih Rabbani

~~~

Such work as homemaking, child rearing, running a home-based business, or leaving the home to go to a place of employment are essential aspects of being a healthy human being. When you do work in a spirit of service to others, it is highly fulfilling and a way of serving God.

Of course, work can include stresses. It tests and strengthens character qualities like patience, perseverance, self-discipline, honesty, trustworthiness, and many more. Learning to interact cooperatively with others is one of the most difficult efforts you will make in life. Work builds skills, talents, and capacity for being strong in all of life's adventures.

Couples often help each other with their work issues through listening, problem-solving, and encouraging. It's wise and important for both of you to express appreciation to the other for your efforts and sacrifices toward your family and financial support. There is a balance, however. If you put so much energy and time toward home, children, or paid employment that you neglect each other, your couple well-being will suffer. Part of the balance can be showing interest and becoming involved in what each other is doing. You may also make new choices for how you spend your time.

**A Couple's Experience:**

*"We each work outside our home, and one of us also has a part-time home-based business. We often arrive home very tired and with multiple family responsibilities to handle once we get there. As we have assessed what is not working for us in this situation, we have begun to make some changes.*

*"One of us is choosing a new work position that will allow for leaving our home an hour later in the mornings. On the weekend, we make some meals ahead for the week. We are asking our children to take on more responsibility. We alternate who gets exercise time in the mornings or evenings. And we are sharing the home-based business responsibilities to increase time together on a common activity."*

**Well-Being Discussion:**

- How do we view and feel about our work? How does our work benefit others?
- How do we, or could we, help each other with our work? How does our example of working affect our children?
- How do we view our current work/life balance? What do we want to do differently?

**Learning Activities to Try:**

- At the end of the day, share three things we are grateful for from our work that day.
- Identify a problem that is occurring in each of our work situations, consult with each other to build understanding, and strategize potential solutions.
- Assess work responsibilities of all types and develop ways for reducing or delegating some of them.

**Conscious Focus:**

"We work productively to support ourselves and our family, and we consider our family when making work and time choices."

## 15 - MONEY

**Reflections:**

"Where money intersects most deeply with our emotions is a complex and vulnerable place. Money, like nothing else we know of, is the screen on which couples project all their deepest fears, hopes, dreams, and hurts in life. You can learn a lot about your relationship and the deeper longings of each other's hearts if you are able to understand what money symbolizes. ... All couples have money problems, and even the happiest couples don't ever solve some of their key money problems... There are many things that go into great solutions. Two of the most important are teamwork and patience. When making the bigger decisions in life, couples who make the best solutions, the solutions most likely to last, go slowly but hand in hand. ... When you settle prematurely on a solution, you are likely to pay for the lack of planning with more conflict eruption about the issue later on."[38] N. Jenkins, S. Stanley, W. Bailey, and H. Markman

"True we must work hard, earn money and keep our family in happiness and prosperity, but we must always realize that our lives must be devoted to things higher and more sublime."[39] On behalf of Shoghi Effendi

~~~

Money is one of the most complex issues couples deal with. Discussions arise about who earns it, who manages it, how to save it or invest it, what it gets spent on and when, whether going into debt makes sense, how to support family members, how to teach children financial responsibility, and more. Each person has their own history of experiences related to money, and the blend of both of your experiences can result in very different approaches and viewpoints. Flexibility, creativity, and a focus on finding harmonious solutions are all vital not only for peace but for the prosperity of the family.

Being without enough money for necessities presents one set of challenges. Having a lot of money can bring a different set to manage. It's wise to determine what is essential and necessary for your lives. Then you can see whether to increase income or whether you have money to spend on non-necessities. If you find that you are spending a great deal of time trying to manage your money, you may choose to hire others to help.

Money can aid your physical well-being through improved nutrition, access to exercise facilities, and so on. Money can also more importantly open opportunities to your family to carry out what you value, such as pursuing an education, traveling to serve others, and maintaining a healthy and welcoming home.

Money management also includes concepts like sacrifice, thriftiness, and generosity. When you are good stewards of the money you have, it builds self-respect and couple respect. As you conserve your resources, you are more able to be generous in sharing them with others. Then you agree between you or as a family who and what entities you give to. From a spiritual standpoint, couples will consult about how and how much they assist the funds and activities that match their beliefs.

**A Couple's Experience:**

*"We didn't know when we became a couple which of us would manage our funds and what would be kept separate and what would be joined. We began with a mix of both and observed what turned out well and what didn't.*

*"It has evolved that the one who is working at home is better with managing the mail and bills. Over time, there has also been more joining of funds and less kept separate. We regularly consult with each other and with a financial planner about how to manage our money and where to make sacrifices in support of family members. We also consult as a family about what money goes to charity and the Bahá'í Faith's various funds."*

**Well-Being Discussion:**

- What did our family experiences teach us about money as we were growing up?
- What are we saving toward and why? What are our children saving toward and why?
- When are we able to be thrifty? Generous with family, friends, or charities?

**Learning Activities to Try:**

- Determine when it's important to each other to discuss and agree on an expenditure before it happens, considering what types of items we might want to purchase and what amounts would be reasonable to spend.
- Write down a plan for where we want to be financially in 5 years, 10 years, and 25 years and strategize about how we will get there.
- Identify a charity that we want to give money to and how much and how often we will donate.

**Conscious Focus:**

"Money is a valuable resource that benefits us, our family, and others."

## 16 - COMMUNICATION

**Reflections:**

"Content, volume, style, tact, wisdom, timeliness are among the critical factors in determining the effects of speech for good or evil. Consequently, the friends need ever to be conscious of the significance of this activity which so distinguishes human beings from other forms of life, and they must exercise it judiciously. Their efforts at such discipline will give birth to an etiquette of expression worthy of the approaching maturity of the human race. Just as this discipline applies to the spoken word, it applies equally to the written word…."[40] Universal House of Justice

"When your dialogue feels safe, loving, and satisfying, your relationship feels like a good one. If talking together becomes dominating, tense, rude, or bruising, the relationship feels both less secure and less appealing. Moreover, since verbal interaction occurs during so much of the time you spend together, and is essential to the business of living together, how you talk to each other becomes the single best indicator of the health of your relationship."[41] Susan Heitler, PhD

~~~

    The quality of your communications has a direct effect on you as individuals and on your ability to be trusted companions with each other. The interactions your children see affect their security, feelings of safety, and well-being. Your communications and actions are important ways of conveying love and appreciation. Often you will speak to one another, but you also connect with words and graphics by various electronic means, such as text messages, social media, or email. You also share photographs and quotations that send a message.
    Your facial expressions, tone of voice, and body language all convey information to each other and to your children. It's wise to be very conscious about what you are intending to communicate

and the best way to share that message. It's difficult to maintain couple and family well-being if you are constantly dealing with misunderstandings, hurt feelings, assumptions, reactions, and more.

While it's important for both of you to be responsible for what you communicate and how, no one can achieve complete clarity and be fully understood every time. As you send and receive communications, part of what you use your words for is to check for understanding as needed. When it's important for your relationship, it's wise to clarify what the speaker meant. Go back and forth, summarizing what you heard and asking gentle questions, until you understand each other.

When you have something difficult to communicate with each other, pay attention to whether it's a good time and place. Do you need alone time first? Do you both need to eat or sleep first? Sometimes it can be useful to engage in some positive action before and after sharing. This might include sharing an appreciation for something the other did, offering a prayer, or giving a hug. You will learn over time what is best for each of you.

**A Couple's Experience:**

*"We have both lived in homes where communication was painful, frustrating, and angry. We never knew whether our partners were being truthful. We were determined to not be together if that was going to be the culture of our relationship. With many experiences over time, we learned that we both prefer to approach our interactions with timeliness, truthfulness, and love. The combination has us fully share what's on our minds and hearts. We soften the edges with kindness, and often humor as well.*

*"We stay very conscious about limiting communications between us when either of us is hungry, overly tired, angry, distracted with major projects, or not feeling well. It helps us communicate well when we recognize that we highly value our relationship, and so we want to protect it from harm."*

**Well-Being Discussion:**

- What are our favorite types of communication? What can we do to prevent hurtful communications?
- What can we do to ensure we are paying attention to each other and not distracted when communications need to happen?
- Are we generally able to control the volume of our voices and apply tact and kindness for successful communications? Where can we improve?

**Learning Activities to Try:**

- Study a book or articles on couple communication together; watch videos on the topic; begin practicing one or two new ways of interacting.
- Set a time to give each other focused attention and discuss issues of importance (one at a time) to each of using tactfulness, truthfulness, and wisdom.
- Practice two new ways of communicating love and appreciation with each other for a week. Include the children as appropriate.

**Conscious Focus:**

"We use communication to convey important thoughts and feelings in ways that we both enjoy."

## 17 - LISTENING

**Reflections:**

"*Good* communication means having the impact you intended to have, that is, Intent equals Impact. In other words, good communication between intimates is clear and precise. The speaker tries to clarify the intent of his message by stating exactly what he is thinking, wanting, or feeling. He does not assume the listener 'knows' what is going on in his head; he tells the listener so that the listener doesn't have to guess or mind read. The good listener tries to make sure that the intent of the message is understood, and does not fill in gaps with guesses as to what is going on in the speaker's mind. Both partners are trying to make sure that Intent equals Impact."[42] J. Gottman, C. Notarius, J. Gonso, and H. Markman

"To the questioner He responded first with silence—an outward silence. His encouragement always was that the other should speak and He listen. There was never that eager tenseness, that restlessness so often met showing most plainly that the listener has the pat answer ready the moment he should have a chance to utter it.

"I have heard certain people described as 'good listeners', but never had I imagined such a 'listener' as 'Abdu'l-Bahá. It was more than a sympathetic absorption of what the ear received. It was as though the two individualities became one; as if He so closely identified Himself with the one speaking that a merging of spirits occurred which made a verbal response almost unnecessary, superfluous. As I write, the words of Bahá'u'lláh recur to me: 'When the sincere servant calls to Me in prayer I become the very ear with which he heareth My reply.'

"That was just it! 'Abdu'l-Bahá seemed to listen with my ears."[43] Howard Colby Ives

~~~

Some people think it's romantic to believe that your true love can (and should!) "read your mind". In this scenario, there is no reason to clearly communicate or spend time listening. It's best to leave mind-reading for fiction. The gift of your listening to each other is one way of showing generosity and love. It lets each other know that you care, and you want to understand. It's a way to bring your minds and hearts closer in unity.

Being effective at listening takes practice. It includes being able to focus on what each other is saying rather than getting sidetracked into formulating a response or trying to come up with a solution. With careful listening, you become aware of more than the words. From tone of voice and body language, as well as the words, you can tune into each other's unmet needs or unexpressed feelings. As you check for understanding, include gentle inquiries about these. Some people don't really know what they are thinking and feeling until they are encouraged to say something out loud. If you are good listeners and can encourage each other to fully share, you will build understanding much better.

You will be most effective with listening if you arrange your bodies and environment in a way that assists with connection. For children, you may need to lower yourselves to their level. With each other, it can be useful to go for a walk or arrange chairs side-by-side or facing each other.

**A Couple's Experience:**

*"One aspect I appreciate most in my partner's listening is his ability to step away from defensiveness and step into my world with gentle questions and listening. I watch his conscious self-control and choice to not react. Instead he stretches to understand what I'm saying. It helps, too, that we are both open to explore the actions we each took that contributed to the problem under discussion."*

**Well-Being Discussion:**

- What do we consider as each other's strengths with listening?

- What would contribute to us listening to each other better?
- How can we integrate effective listening into our daily lives?

**Learning Activities to Try:**

- Set a certain time with no use of technology, such as phones or computers, and engage in talking and listening with each other about something important to both of us.
- Choose a current issue and practice listening for and clarifying the wants and needs each other is feeling but may not be fully expressing.
- Share a story from childhood and have the other summarize the story and what they observed about the situation and the feelings involved; take turns.

**Conscious Focus:**

"We listen to understand each other's mind, heart, and soul."

## 18 - APPRECIATION

**Reflections:**

"We can never exert the influence over others which we can exert over ourselves. If we are better, if we show love, patience, and understanding of the weakness of others, if we seek to never criticize but rather encourage, others will do likewise…."[44] Shoghi Effendi

"*Appreciation* is an expression of pleasure from the speaker's point of view. The message is 'I value (like, enjoy) what you did.' Appreciation is easy to communicate and rewarding to receive. Appreciation is commonly used by many people, so it is familiar. Appreciation tells another person that his or her deed was noticed and it benefited the speaker. Appreciation can motivate a partner to repeat the behavior…."[45] Sandra Gray Bender, PhD

~~~

It can be easy to assume that people close to you know what you appreciate about them and their actions, especially when you get busy and don't express the words to them. However, there is tremendous power to touch the heart of another person through offering sincere and kind words of appreciation and encouragement. This is effective even when an action is one the other does often.

Daily tasks like cooking and washing the dishes are easier to accomplish when someone notices and thanks you for doing them well. Hearing how delicious a meal is, encourages the person who cooked to do it again and to be creative with their efforts. Expressing appreciation to your children encourages them to keep striving in service to the family or with their school or work tasks.

When you sacrifice time for each other or do extra very thoughtful actions, appreciation is especially important. Marshall Rosenberg, author of *Nonviolent Communication: A Language of Life* (p. 186), encourages expressions of appreciation when someone has contributed to your well-being, when they have fulfilled a need, and when there are feelings of pleasure with the meeting of those needs.

In an intimate relationship, even simply saying "thank you" and linking it to something specific can have a powerful positive effect. Your partner will be more likely to repeat the positive action. Appreciation lets each other know that you see each other, you notice what each other is doing, and you honor the effect of each other's actions in your life.

Pay attention to how you each respond to words of appreciation and encouragement from each other:

- Does your ego get triggered, and you think you are now better than the other?
- Do you struggle with low self-respect, and discount each other's positive words?
- Are you able to accept the words with joy and be happy your partner appreciated your actions?

When you are both emotionally healthy, and you focus on expressing gratitude for each other's actions, appreciative and encouraging words build love, connection, and couple well-being.

## A Couple's Experience:

*"I have found that when my stress level starts to rise, it almost immediately triggers resentment that family members are not valuing my contributions. I feel like I need to call special attention to the things I am doing. We have noticed that stress also prevents me from seeing the contributions that others are making, and so I miss opportunities to express appreciation. Both of us make an effort now to say or show our appreciation for each other whenever we can, but especially in times of stress."*

**Well-Being Discussion:**

- How are we showing our respect and appreciation for each other's accomplishments?
- How do we respond to encouragement from one another?
- What do we notice each other doing every day that we rarely express appreciation for? What can we say or do now to express appreciation for these? How does it feel to receive appreciation?

**Learning Activities to Try:**

- Make a list(s) of what we appreciate about each other; when we think about criticizing each other, read the appreciation list(s) and notice how that shifts our perspectives.
- Write a letter of appreciation to someone who has contributed to our relationship.
- Try using *Character Quality Language*™, where you acknowledge each other through specifically and sincerely using character qualities in your appreciations. This encouraging practice touches hearts, builds character and relationships, and brings happiness. Here are some simple examples:

    - "Thank you for being (Helpful, Flexible, Truthful…) when you…."
    - "I appreciated your (Courage, Respect, Patience…) when you…"
    - "I love how (Accepting, Enthusiastic, Encouraging…) you are!"

**Conscious Focus:**

"We do our best to notice and appreciate the best in each other and in each other's actions, and we celebrate each other's accomplishments."

## 19 - FEELINGS

**Reflections:**

"... [W]hat others say and do may be the stimulus, but never the cause, of our feelings. We see that our feelings result from how we choose to receive what others say and do, as well as from our particular needs and expectations in that moment. ... [W]e are led to accept responsibility for what we do to generate our own feelings."[46] Marshall B. Rosenberg, PhD

"... [T]he function of language is to portray the mysteries and secrets of human hearts. The heart is like a box, and language is the key. Only by using the key can we open the box and observe the gems it contains."[47] 'Abdu'l-Bahá

~~~

The diversity and range of your feelings adds color, flavor, and complex and interesting layers to your lives. Sometimes feelings seem positive, and at other times very uncomfortable or even destructive. It's an ongoing learning experience to determine how to understand and express your feelings in constructive ways.

Sometimes you may need time alone to assess, understand, and accept what you are feeling and why. Sometimes you decide what happened was minor. Yet other times, it takes physical action to release strong emotions such as anger. Some people find release by cleaning the house, building something that requires hammering, going for a brisk walk, hitting a punching bag, or scribbling on a large piece of paper with black and red markers. What is vital is determining how to handle the feelings without harming each other.

After reflection and the calming of emotions, then it may make sense to share thoughts and feelings with each other. This sharing can help you sort out what is happening.

It enriches the lives of couples and families when you expand your vocabulary of words that describe feelings. Some people can only label happy, sad, and angry in themselves. You can be more specific and increase understanding if you share that you are feeling such emotions as: frustrated, scared, safe, curious, excited, delighted, satisfied, serene, relieved, amazed, hopeful, astonished, concerned, and more.

When you focus on discussing an issue and determining solutions, sharing what you are feeling can contribute to deeper understanding. When you understand how the issue or solution affects each other emotionally, you can make more effective couple decisions.

**A Couple's Experience:**

*"When I feel really frustrated, I have to find something to clean or organize. Acting this way helps my mind calm down and my thoughts be more orderly. Often it becomes clear that I was being judgmental, and when I am calmer, I become more reasonable. It's easier to see someone else's point of view. When we then discuss the issue, I share how frustrated I was as well as my changed perspectives. Then we can move into problem-solving consultation together."*

**Well-Being Discussion:**

- What positive feelings connect us to each other? What could increase these positive feelings?
- How can we constructively release negative feelings?
- How could it benefit our relationship and family if we expand our vocabulary of feelings?

**Learning Activities to Try:**

- Pick three new words that describe our feelings and include them in daily conversations.
- Try out a new way of releasing negative feelings.
- Identify one or two unmet needs that are leading to uncomfortable feelings and take steps to address the needs.

**Conscious Focus:**

"We honor the full range of feelings we have that enrich our lives, and we encourage each other to express them in ways that enhance our well-being."

## 20 - DECISIONS

**Reflections:**

"... [T]he rights of each and all in the family unit must be upheld, ...loving consultation should be the keynote, ...all matters must be settled in harmony and love... [T]here are times when the husband and the wife should defer to the wishes of the other. Exactly under what circumstances such deference should take place is a matter for each couple to determine. If...they fail to agree, and their disagreement leads to estrangement, they should seek counsel from those they trust and in whose sincerity and sound judgment they have confidence, in order to preserve and strengthen their ties as a united family."[48] On behalf of the Universal House of Justice

"The tone of collaborative dialogue is friendly. Even when the topic is a serious one, the tone still feels cooperative, as if you have placed your problem on a table and the two of you have sat down side by side to try to solve it. You feel that you are confronting the problem together, rather than that you are confronting each other.
"Another tip-off that dialogue is collaborative is that you feel a sense of forward movement as you accumulate shared understanding. Adversarial dialogue feels repetitive. When dialogue is cooperative, with each successive comment you feel movement toward a shared plan of action."[49] Susan Heitler, PhD

~~~

Unity is vital in maintaining healthy and happy relationships, and it's often the *means* to solving problems and reaching agreements. When you are committed to moving forward together, unified decision-making increases your harmony by aligning your values and intentions over time. You share your thoughts, feelings, wishes, and dreams.

When you have discussions for building understanding and solving problems, you are not attached at the beginning to a particular outcome. Instead, you are open to a creative exchange of ideas, thoughts, and feelings so you achieve a better solution together. When one of you doesn't have a strong opinion about a solution, or one of you has special expertise, it can occasionally make sense to defer to the other. However, you are still united in supporting the efforts and outcomes.

Unity helps you effectively carry out any decisions you make. When you value unity, you consciously look for points of agreement, harmony, and attraction. You collaborate as partners in building a strong foundation of oneness, love, commitment, and cooperation. Unity is not sameness—rather, it is honoring the idea that you both bring diverse perspectives and unique approaches to your couple consultations. You respect how these differing views enhance potential solutions.

When you are united, you feel and act as if you are on the same team, and you demonstrate a spirit of goodwill toward each other. You know that what you create together is better than anything you could create separately.

**A Couple's Experience:**

*"We had a difficult and complicated decision to make about whether to sell property where our friends were renting a home. We had to determine what promises had been made to them and how the sale money could benefit our family members. We were concerned about maintaining the friendship if the sale forced the friends to move. Every time we attempted to consult about the issue, emotions ran high and disunity arose.*

*"We set the matter aside again and again until we were calmer. Finally, we realized we were stuck because we had not involved our friends in the consultation. It only took one evening together with them involved to come to a unified decision, when we had been trying to resolve it for weeks on our own."*

**Well-Being Discussion:**

- What environments, approaches, preparation, and more support us to build understanding and reach unified decisions?

- What helps us achieve high-quality decisions?
- What makes it easier to carry out decisions in unity?

**Learning Activities to Try:**

- Set a time each week to meet (as a couple and/or as a family) and consult about any issues and proceed with making any necessary decisions at that time or in another session.
- Make a list of activities to do as a break, when one is needed during a discussion because disunity is becoming an issue.
- Put a bowl between us as a visual receptacle for each of our contributions to the discussion to help us detach from our own ideas and create the best outcome together.

**Conscious Focus:**

"We are committed to maintaining unity in our relationship and achieving unity through making decisions as equal partners."

## 21 - HUMOR

**Reflections:**

"It is good to laugh. Laughter is a spiritual relaxation. When [we] were in prison [for religious persecution] ...and under the utmost deprivation and difficulties, each of [us] at the close of the day would relate the most ludicrous event which had happened. Sometimes it was a little difficult to find one but always [we] would laugh until the tears would roll down [our] cheeks. Happiness...is never dependent upon material surroundings, otherwise how sad those years would have been. As it was [we] were always in the utmost state of joy and happiness."[50] Howard Colby Ives recalling the words of 'Abdu'l-Bahá

"... [W]hile laughter should not be suppressed or frowned upon, it should not be indulged in at the expense of the feelings of others. What one says or does in a humorous vein should not give rise to prejudice of any kind. You may recall 'Abdu'l-Bahá's caution 'Beware lest ye offend the feelings of anyone, or sadden the heart of any person...' (*Tablets of 'Abdu'l-Bahá, Vol. 1*, p. 45)."[51] On behalf of the Universal House of Justice

"Laughter is a spiritual practice. ... The transformative nature of any spiritual discipline comes with regular practice. When done consistently, it can eventually change our lives. If we make time to invite joy into our lives each day, we will become more aware of joy and laughter in our lives and in the world. Eventually, laughter will become an innate part of who we are."[52] Susan Sparks

~~~

Humor can have many aspects that contribute to well-being in your relationship and family: laughter, smiling, affectionate teasing, banter, jokes, funny stories, playfulness, happiness, joy, and sincere enjoyment of activities. Your ability to lighten up can help you prevent conflict, relax, cope with a difficulty, manage a difficult task, experience gratitude, navigate change, and draw you closer together. It can foster honest emotional intimacy. You can interact with each other's personalities and quirks with fun instead of criticism.

One challenge with humor is that people can misuse it. Sarcasm, ridicule, tromping on feelings, personal put-downs, prejudice, and more cause harm rather than produce joy and love. In addition, each person finds different things funny at times. One of you may laugh, and the other is baffled and does not get the joke at all. Sometimes you may use humor as a shield to avoid revealing your true feelings. The other person may then miss your point or not take it seriously. It takes courage to be more direct and not hide behind a laugh.

It's good to go on a quest to find what prompts you both to lighten up—at the appropriate times and in the best places.

**A Couple's Experience:**

*"When we began living together, every time I left the room for a minute, my marriage partner would turn the light off. I'd go back into the room in darkness, which was very annoying. I realized their need to conserve electricity could be a source of regular conflict. Instead, we became playful about it. Sometimes I turn the light off when my partner is still in a room. There is teasing about whether anxiousness is arising when a light is left on unnecessarily. We joke about whether we can see in the dark. We now own amazing flashlights. Being 'light' about this has become an unexpected source of fun."*

**Well-Being Discussion:**

- When are we playful with one another? How do we respond to physical humor? To intellectual humor?
- When has laughter connected us? When has it contributed to us feeling more confident and secure in our relationship?
- What activities might prompt us to laugh more and feel more connected together?

**Learning Activities to Try:**

- Find and share a video with each other that we both find humorous.
- Share a story from a recent (or childhood) experience that was funny.
- Respond with humor and playfulness to a quirky way we each handle something.

**Conscious Focus:**

"We use humor in a positive way, including actively finding ways to prompt each other's laughter."

## 22 - NATURE

**Reflections:**

"Man, possessed of an inner faculty which plants and animals do not have, a power which enables him to discover the secrets of nature and gain mastery over the environment, has a special responsibility to use his God-given powers for positive ends."[53] On behalf of the Universal House of Justice

"What is that mystery underlying human life which gives to events and to persons the power of...transformation? If one had never before seen a seed, nor heard of its latent life, how difficult to believe that only the cold earth, the warm sun, the descending showers, and the gardener's care were needed to cause its miraculous transformation into the growing form, the budding beauty, the intoxicating fragrance of the rose!"[54] Howard Colby Ives

~~~

It often enhances well-being when you are around what is living and growing. If you seek out nature that is also beautiful, that "calls to your soul", you feel even better. If you both enjoy the experience together, the positive effect increases even more. Sunshine in moderation helps the health of your bones and liver, as well as uplifting your spirits.

Observing storms can assist you to release negative thoughts and build energy. Seeing and smelling beautiful flowers excites your senses and brings joy. Experiencing the changes of weather and seasons shifts your perceptions of life. Immersing yourselves in water is sensuous and relaxing. Spotting beautiful birds and growing animals brings excited smiles.

When your lives are feeling out of balance and your energy depleted, ensuring you spend some time out in nature can restore you. This is true whether you are generally healthy or ill. Outdoors can also be a great place for exercise: walking, biking, kayaking, swimming, and much more. You can stretch and tone muscles, rebalance your minds, and generate endorphins, those hormones that make you feel good.

**A Couple's Experience:**

*"We get up most mornings, say prayers, and then go out for a two-mile walk. The joy and calm of the prayers follow us, and consultation is always best at these times. We are fresh and alone, and the presence of God abounds. We feel united in our love and intentions, and we consult about how we can help make each other's day smoother.*

*"When we were dealing with a big issue, we needed a big space for consulting, and so we did most of it on walks outside. This gave each of us the chance to say what we needed to say. We had the space and distance to process our feelings and consider our options and responses without having to immediately speak. We were surrounded by nature and by God, and it gave us privacy."*

**Well-Being Discussion:**

- What types of nature experiences most appeal to us? How do we respond to spending time in nature together?
- What actions can we take to protect the environment?
- How can we bring nature into our home environment?

**Learning Activities to Try:**

- Find a new park in your area and spend the day there.
- Rent a boat or other watercraft and spend time on the water, watching the sunset together if possible.
- Take an action that benefits the environment.

**Conscious Focus:**

"We look for opportunities to be together in nature."

## 23 - CREATIVITY

**Reflections:**

"All created things are expressions of the affinity and cohesion of elementary substances, and non-existence is the absence of their attraction and agreement. Various elements unite harmoniously in composition but when these elements become discordant, repelling each other, decomposition and non-existence result. Everything partakes of this nature and is subject to this principle, for the creative foundation in all its degrees and kingdoms is an expression or outcome of love."[55] 'Abdu'l-Bahá

"True creativity often starts where language ends."[56] Arthur Koestler

~~~

When you have ways of expressing yourselves creatively, without feeling a need to achieve perfection, you feel a flow of energy rise in you and outward into action. Encouragement and appreciation from each other often increase this creativity. Many people feel they aren't creative at all and have no ability to be so. However, this is an innate quality in everyone. How you express it might simply need a broader definition.

For some people, creativity only looks like art, music, design, or crafts. It's often an inner imperative for them to create in these ways. In addition, creativity can take many other forms. Perhaps it is the way you decorate your home. Maybe it is how you approach a home repair. You could be creative in how you mix ingredients together for a meal. The way you lay out flowers in your garden or arrange them in a vase could express your creativity.

Creativity links to inspiration, being open to new ideas and concepts. Some people use meditation or prayer to help. Some people put themselves in what they consider a creative environment, such as an art museum or garden. Whatever your source of inspiration, it's essential to recognize that creative expressions usually increase your sense of well-being.

Expressing yourself creatively increases your self-respect, expands your vision, and produces beauty, however you define that. When you share with each other what you have created, it becomes a couple-unifying experience.

**A Couple's Experience:**

*"We are both creative in different ways. One of us is excellent at 'shade-tree engineering', which economically solves a repair challenge or problem in unique ways with a mix of objects. The other takes beautiful photographs and shares them with others. We both appreciate what the other does."*

**Well-Being Discussion:**

- What does creativity look like to us?
- Which creative expressions are happy and positive? Which ones are more likely to feel stressful?
- Would we need to do something "useful" with what we create for it to feel valuable?

**Learning Activities to Try:**

- Visit a hardware, furniture, or crafts store and explore ideas of creative expressions and home decorations.
- Purchase food ingredients and create a new meal together.
- Try an arts activity, such as painting, coloring, photography, a craft, composing a song, or writing a poem, either together or separately. If the activity is done separately, then share the outcome together.

**Conscious Focus:**

"We love the exhilaration of releasing creative energy."

## 24 - RESILIENCE

**Reflections:**

"Studies show that resilient people—those who are able to cope with adversity and bounce back from stressful experiences quickly and efficiently—have three distinguishing characteristics: an acceptance of reality, a strongly held belief that life is meaningful, and an ability to find creative solutions to seemingly insoluble problems."[57] Janet A. Khan

"Courage is love as action—love on her silver steed, forcing change in the world, rising to challenges, negotiating life with skill, and confronting others with care and wisdom. The qualities that courage draws upon—hardiness and resilience, as well as the ability to bend and alter course when faced with difficulty, to commit oneself to a cause, and to find inner power during times of pain—are *all* associated with mental health. We need a deep, tensile strength to face the tough times in life, to speak out persuasively against injustice, and, above all, to love others wisely and well. To love at all is a risk that requires courage—we risk our safety, letting ourselves be raw and vulnerable; we accept our share of compromise and weather disappointment and despair; and above all, we are willing to confront a loved one even if what we need to say is not easy or kind."[58] Stephen Post

~~~

    Your individual, couple, and family well-being is dependent upon your ability to find your way back from difficult experiences, mistakes, or illnesses. You are partners in this process of finding balance again, or at least a "new normal". Together you will clarify your goal—where you want to reach in your efforts. Then you will make a plan and take action. Your perseverance and determination will move you in a positive direction.
    When you are resilient, you accept and adjust to changing circumstances instead of whining, complaining, and grumbling

about them. You assess your strengths and resources and focus them on bouncing back instead of staying stuck in a poor situation. You do your best to improve on situations and move yourselves back toward well-being.

**A Couple's Experience:**

*"My marriage partner was regularly verbally criticized or undermined at work, although often in subtle and manipulative ways. Daily life was filled with vulnerability, being on guard, resistance to working near the difficult fellow employee, and more. Eventually there was a serious incident, resulting in an appeal for managerial help, and illness struck. Then I got sick too. The illness got stuck in our home and didn't want to leave. We had to find an alternative medical practitioner who could address both the emotional root causes and the physical symptoms. Then we could both begin to bounce back and move on."*

**Well-Being Discussion:**

- What helps us recover from making a mistake or hurting each other's feelings?
- How do we respond to problems and move forward from them?
- When have we found working cooperatively on an issue increased our resilience?

**Learning Activities to Try:**

- Check in with each other daily or regularly to see if there is anything to "clean up" that caused a problem between us.
- Identify something that needs focused attention for recovery.
- Play a game that involves recovering from losses and making gains.

**Conscious Focus:**

"We maintain our relationship harmony and well-being by addressing issues on a timely basis and seeking effective recovery and resolution."

## 25 - RESOURCEFULNESS

**Reflections:**

"See difficulties as learning opportunities that will expand your talents and capacities. Remind yourself that you can positively influence much of what happens in life. See yourself as capable and as an active participant in your world. Even when a problem has aspects that cannot be changed, trust that if you are resourceful, you will be able to use the situation to learn new ways of responding to it. Welcome change and challenge. Have faith that greater life meaning and satisfaction will emerge from each stressful situation."[59] Stephen Post

"... [L]ive a selfless life of service and use your resources for the betterment of the world. Consort in fellowship and work with all who strive for these noble aims."[60] Universal House of Justice

"Consultation is...available for the individual in solving his own problems; he may consult with his Assembly, with his family and with his friends."[61] On behalf of the Universal House of Justice; *Note: A Spiritual Assembly is an elected council in the Bahá'í Faith.*

~~~

Couples and families benefit from having a good support system. Key well-being skills are being resourceful in learning and in gathering help before you need it and drawing on it when you do. Your support team could include the following and more:

- Healthy couples
- Family members
- Friends
- Financial professionals
- Medical personnel
- Counsellors
- Spiritual or religious services
- Support groups
- Parenting experts
- Nutritionists
- Legal help

- Exercise coaches and trainers
- Self-help books
- Neighbors

It takes some humility to admit that you often cannot maintain your optimum well-being on your own, but it's very true.

Generally, people are happy when you ask them for assistance, and they are helpful in response. However, as you build the resources you need for support, pause to observe whether someone is contributing positively to your lives or not. Sometimes it's best to "uninvite" people from your team and replace them with someone new. Building and maintaining a support team is an organic process that adjusts as your needs change.

**A Couple's Experience:**

*"We began to look ahead to make some new choices in our lives. We wanted to increase our savings so that we could be freer to travel as a family and offer services to others at times. We were a bit concerned about our general health and well-being. We wanted to add on to our home, so we had a room for children's classes and youth to gather, as well as a guest room to make it easier for grandparents to visit.*

*"We decided to invite two other couples in our age range and similar circumstances to come consult with us. Together we made specific plans to address these issues. The other couples benefited from seeing ways to improve their lives as well."*

**Well-Being Discussion:**

- Who do we consider part of our support team?
- What support do we need occasionally? What is helpful for addressing an ongoing need?
- Where could we benefit from expanding our support network? Who could we ask?

**Learning Activities to Try:**

- Make a contact list of the people we consider effective resources for us. Identify and reach out to a new resource person.
- Have dinner out with a happy, healthy couple or invite a happy, healthy family to our home.
- Identify a new learning resource for us (book, course, videos...) that will strengthen our relationship and well-being.

**Conscious Focus:**

"We are resourceful in building a support team of people who help us as needed and requested."

## 26 - SPIRITUALITY

**Reflections:**

"… [S]pirituality is the greatest of God's gifts, and 'Life Everlasting' means 'Turning to God.' May you, one and all, increase daily in spirituality, may you be strengthened in all goodness, may you be helped more and more by the Divine consolation, be made free by the Holy Spirit of God, and may the power of the Heavenly Kingdom live and work among you."[62] 'Abdu'l-Bahá

"Authentic spirituality means giving up perfectionism for the rigorous process of developing ourselves one thought, one act, one day at a time."[63] Linda Kavelin Popov

~~~

You each have your own ways of connecting to spiritual sources and expressing spirituality in your lives. You might believe in God or a Higher Power. You may follow a religious faith or set of beliefs, separately or together. Perhaps prayer and meditation are practices in your life, as these are significant ways to cultivate a sense of spirituality. Perhaps you worship with others.

Spiritual practices can have significant power in maintaining your balance and well-being. When you can mutually participate in some of those practices, the connection between you deepens and strengthens.

You become more centered and calmer when you spend time in reflection and meditation, connect to a Power greater than you, and nurture your soul. Spirituality empowers your ability to gradually transform your words and actions. When you seek help and wisdom from inspirational sources, your knowledge, character, and positive behaviors expand and grow. As you express gratitude for blessings and ask for help with challenges, you humbly admit you don't have all the answers. Inviting spiritual influences into your life together links you in a powerful way.

**A Couple's Experience:**

*"We decided to see if it would make a difference in our relationship if we began to pray together. It was easy to put it into our routine during the week, and it seemed to draw us closer together. We even prayed together on the phone when we were apart. During unstructured weekends, it was more difficult. What we noticed, however, was that we were far more likely to be critical of each other or annoyed with the other's behaviors on the days we did not pray. When we did pray together, it was easier to see the best in each other and strive for unity and harmony."*

**Well-Being Discussion:**

- How can we express and practice spirituality or our religious beliefs in our lives in ways that build unity between us and between us and others?
- How does spiritual well-being contribute to us? Our family?
- How do we draw on spiritual resources to foster personal growth, such as applying kindness and compassion?

**Learning Activities to Try:**

- Practice praying and/or meditating together and not praying and/or meditating together and see what contributions these actions make in our relationship.
- Plan and carry out a devotional gathering where there are prayers and spiritual readings.
- Participate in the worship services of our faith paths.

**Conscious Focus:**

"We draw on spirituality to strengthen our connection, unity, and well-being."

## 27 - SERVICE

**Reflections:**

"The call to carry out and support this work [of community building] is directed to every follower of Bahá'u'lláh, and it will evoke a response in every heart that aches at the wretched condition of the world, the lamentable circumstances from which so many people are unable to gain relief. For, ultimately, it is systematic, determined, and selfless action undertaken within the wide embrace of... [a global plan] that is the most constructive response of every concerned believer to the multiplying ills of a disordered society."[64] Universal House of Justice

"Living to promote the betterment of others and of humanity as a whole is part and parcel of the purpose of life. The purpose of finding a partner is not to be free of loneliness or to enjoy the thrills of falling in love, rather, it is to find someone who will be an intimate partner in our path of service and one with whom we can have children who will also be reared in an attitude of serving the good of humanity. A worthy goal of loving and building a life together is to contribute to the betterment of the world."[65] Raymond Switzer

~~~

    A key aspect of service is to look toward the needs of your marriage and family and ensure that you meet them. Thoughtful service to each other keeps you emotionally connected. The quality of your marriage and family life that includes respect for parents supports your well-being and provides inspiration and encouragement to others. A unified marriage and family provide a building block for a united human family.
    Part of living a balanced life of well-being also includes giving service to others beyond your immediate family. How, where, and why you serve will vary according to your beliefs, passions, interests, and ability to have an impact with your efforts. You can have an outward-looking orientation in your relationship through striving to

understand the reality of your neighborhood or region. You could build friendships with neighbors, sharing hospitality back and forth with them, and having meaningful conversations. You could see a social or structural problem that needs to be addressed in your community, and you then build a cooperative approach to addressing it along with others. You might become involved with children's education or assisting youth. The inward foundation of couple well-being you have built, and that you maintain regularly, gives you the strength to reach out and make a difference for others.

As you consider ways to serve, you might give time or advice to an organization. Maybe you volunteer at your child's school. You might start a new business or organization to meet a need. You might trade or share childcare with other parents. As you look at options, remember that the earlier children and youth engage in service, the more likely it will always be part of their lives.

Service could involve actions that make a difference to one person or a few, perhaps in very personal ways. Alternatively, you might be someone who appreciates creating new systems to meet broader needs. Whatever you choose to do, look for ways the service can also enhance your couple relationship and unity. This may mean taking actions together, or it could be that you consult and create ideas together of actions to do separately. Then you can share insights together after acting.

**A Couple's Experience:**

*"For two months in the summer, we decided to host a weekly picnic in the yard of our home. We invited people from our neighborhood and some other friends and set up games and music. At the beginning, we provided all the food and drinks. However, everyone began to participate and brought their favorite dishes to share.*

*"After a month where we built friendships, we began a serious conversation about an area of our community that was experiencing regular violence. It was clear many were upset about the problem. We began to list some of what we could do to respond to the*

*situation. We felt more hopeful and empowered as people volunteered for the necessary tasks."*

**Well-Being Discussion:**

- How does our marriage integrate with a commitment to have service be a central aspect of our lives?
- How do we feel about reaching out to serve others? How could this build our capacity to be of service within our home and family?
- What types of service appeal to us most? Where could our children best participate?

**Learning Activities to Try:**

- Do a thoughtful act for each other and/or each family member every day for a week and see how it benefits us.
- Talk with people we know who are doing community service about what they are doing and why they are doing it. Consult together about what to get involved in. Take steps to participate.
- Host a group of friends in our home; pray and consult together about what we could do to positively influence the lives of others. Consider starting or hosting a Bahá'í-based spiritual study circle or some other type of outreach activity.

**Conscious Focus:**

"We are happy to contribute the example of our marriage, our time and other resources, and our abilities to others."

## 28 - UNITY

**Reflections:**

"Note ye how easily, where unity existeth in a given family, the affairs of that family are conducted; what progress the members of that family make, how they prosper in the world. Their concerns are in order, they enjoy comfort and tranquility, they are secure, their position is assured, they come to be envied by all. Such a family but addeth to its stature and its lasting honor, as day succeedeth day."[66] 'Abdu'l-Bahá

"A healthy marriage is the union of two individuated, differentiated persons. These are people truly capable of loving the uniqueness of each other. Thus, the union of marriage is not ever intended to be enmeshment or unity in conformity, as this would attenuate who we can truly be. Rather, with unity in diversity, we grow together through a true realization of our wider potential and primal oneness. Mindful differentiation always develops through connection, not disconnection."[67] Raymond and Furugh Switzer

"The world of humanity is possessed of two wings: the male and the female. … When the two wings or parts become equivalent in strength, enjoying the same prerogatives, the flight of man will be exceedingly lofty and extraordinary. Therefore, woman must receive the same education as man and all inequality be adjusted. Thus, imbued with the same virtues as man, rising through all the degrees of human attainment, women will become the peers of men, and until this equality is established, true progress and attainment for the human race will not be facilitated."[68] 'Abdu'l-Bahá

~~~

Healthy couples yearn for and look for opportunities to create unity or oneness. The sense of harmony between you, even though you clearly are different people, is one of the benefits of well-being between you. You look for points of agreement, strive to create unified decisions, and arrange your lives to flow without destructive conflict. You ensure that on balance your lives are fair toward each other. You don't assume that a period of unhappiness is forever, and you keep looking for ways to improve your situation.

The quality of your friendship, your companionship, your enjoyment of each other's company, your mutual respect and equality, all contribute to unity. Your ability to find spiritual connection, your sharing of humorous moments, and your ability to function as a family are all aspects of unity. You are connected, integrated, one. The strength of your couple unity empowers you both to create unity with others.

**A Couple's Experience:**

*"We both went through a number of relationship experiences with others where it was very difficult to maintain unity. Anger, unfaithfulness, immaturity, poor character, and more interfered in being able to feel united. When we found each other, it was like being able to breathe again, and we could breathe together.*

*"When we hold each other or are intimate, it's like being one body. When we consult through a problem, it's like we are one mind. When we express love to one another, it's like we are one heart. When we pray, it's like being one soul."*

**Well-Being Discussion:**

- What contributes toward our unity? Have we arranged our lives in a way that is fair to both of us?
- When do we feel a sense of oneness with each other? With others?
- When we feel disunity begin between us in a discussion, how can we change course?

**Learning Activities to Try:**

- Make a list of 10 points of harmony or agreement between us.

- Make a list of 5 ways we are different, and we appreciate and benefit from the diversity.
- Choose two actions that could increase a feeling of strong connection between us and carry them out.

**Conscious Focus:**

"Maintaining the strength of our union through conscious thought, words, and action is a very high commitment to our well-being."

## **GOAL-SETTING**

**Reminder:** It will be wise for you to have some type of system for setting and keeping track of your specific action goals that arise out of going through this guide and your progress toward these goals. You will be most successful if your goals are clear, agreed-upon, and attainable in a reasonable amount of time.

As you set goals, keep in mind:

- What new actions are we committed to taking in support of our well-being?
- How will we assess our progress?
- When will we review our progress?
- What will we do next?

The rhythm of growth and progress in your marriage, lives, and the community around you is a process of:

- Studying spiritual and scientific information
- Consulting with each other and others
- Acting in alignment with what emerges from the above
- Reflecting on growth, new insights, and possible new directions

Enjoy creating well-being!

## ABOUT THE AUTHOR

Susanne M. Alexander is a Relationship and Marriage Educator and coach, book author, and publisher with Marriage Transformation®:

- www.marriagetransformation.com
- www.transformationlearningcenter.com
- www.bahaimarriages.com

She is certified to offer couple's assessments through Prepare-Enrich and offers individuals the Character Foundations Assessment™. Susanne meets with clients globally via the internet for relationship and marriage preparation and marriage strengthening. Susanne is passionate about accompanying and assisting individuals and couples to make good relationship and marriage choices. Clients build knowledge and skills, something that contributes to healthy relationships and marriages and prevents divorces.

Susanne, a former journalist, writes articles about relationships and marriage for www.bahaiteachings.org and www.bahaiblog.net. She serves as the Department Chair and also as a course developer and faculty member for the Wilmette Institute relationships, marriage, parenting, and family online courses (www.wilmetteinstitute.org).

Susanne has been single, dating, engaged, married, divorced, and widowed. She is a child, stepchild, parent, stepparent, and grandparent. All of this has given Susanne a diversity of experience to share! She is a member of the Bahá'í Faith. Susanne is originally from Canada and is married to a wonderful man in Tennessee, in the United States.

To contact Susanne for her resources and for educational relationship or marriage coaching services, please write to her at susanne@marriagetransformation.com or call/text/WhatsApp at +1 423.599.0153 (US Eastern time zone).

**Disclaimer Note:** Other than the content that is directly from the Bahá'í writings or from another book, the views and perspectives in this book are those of the author.

## ABOUT THE BAHÁ'Í FAITH

For further information about the Bahá'í Faith and those quoted in this book, please access the official international website: www.bahai.org. Many countries also have official websites for their national communities.

## ACKNOWLEDGEMENTS

I extend heartfelt gratitude to an excellent reading team. Your participation was so helpful!

Susanne Alexander

**Reading/Feedback Team:** Rebecca Deerwater, Raven Deerwater, Phil Donihe, Scott Frankowski, Nazanin Heydarian, Ben Imagire, Deidre Imagire, Nikki Lallatin, Marabeth Lum, Rudy Padilla, Alex Sawka, Emily Sawka, Corinne Sheahan, Carly Thaggard, Cecile Wabnitz, Carol Wilhoit, and Johanna Merritt Wu.

# ENDNOTES

[1] Bahá'u'lláh, *Bahá'í Prayers* (US 2002), p. 118
[2] On behalf of Shoghi Effendi, *Compilation of Compilations, Vol. I*, #910
[3] On behalf of the Universal House of Justice, *Lights of Guidance*, #1269
[4] 'Abdu'l-Bahá, *Secret of Divine Civilization*, p. 19
[5] Thomas N. Bradbury, PhD, and Benjamin R. Karney, PhD, *Love Me Slender*, p. 8
[6] W. H. Murray, *Scottish Himalayan Expedition*, pp. 6-7
[7] Martin Seligman, *Authentic Happiness*, p. 8
[8] Shoghi Effendi, *Compilation of Compilations, Vol. I*, #162
[9] On behalf of Shoghi Effendi, "Prayer and Devotional Life" compilation 2019, #10
[10] Shoghi Effendi before he was appointed the Guardian; "The Function of Sport in Life"; http://bahai-library.com/shoghieffendi_function_sports_life
[11] Dan Millman, *Body Mind Mastery*, p. 11
[12] 'Abdu'l-Bahá, *Selections from the Writings of 'Abdu'l-Bahá*, #134
[13] Carl Honoré, *In Praise of Slowness*, p. 58
[14] On behalf of Shoghi Effendi, *Compilation of Compilations, Vol. II*, "Prayer, Meditation and the Devotional Attitude", p. 242
[15] Dale Carnegie, *How to Stop Worrying and Start Living*, p. 24
[16] On behalf of Shoghi Effendi, *Compilation of Compilations, Vol. I*, #1085
[17] Theresa E. DiDonato, PhD, "Why Your Relationship Depends on a Good Night's Sleep", www.psychologytoday.com
[18] 'Abdu'l-Bahá, *Selections from the Writings of 'Abdu'l-Bahá*, #133
[19] Bernie S. Siegel, MD, *Peace, Love, & Healing*, p. 167
[20] Wayne M. Sotile, PhD, and Mary O. Sotile, MA, *Marriage Skills for Busy Couples*, pp. 96; 102; 103
[21] Bahá'u'lláh, *Gleanings from the Writings of Bahá'u'lláh*, p. 216
[22] On behalf of the Universal House of Justice, *Compilation of Compilations, Vol. II*, #2160
[23] 'Abdu'l-Bahá, *Selections from the Writings of 'Abdu'l-Bahá*, #92
[24] John M. Gottman, PhD, and Nan Silver, *Seven Principles for Making Marriage Work* (2nd ed.), pp. 21-22; p. 28
[25] Claudia Arp and David Arp, *10 Great Dates to Energize Your Marriage*, p. 12

26 On behalf of the Universal House of Justice, *Compilation of Compilations, Vol. II*, #2161
27 'Abdu'l-Bahá, *Selections from the Writings of 'Abdu'l-Bahá*, #129
28 Linda Kavelin Popov, *Family Virtues Guide*, p. 73
29 Tim Alan Gardner, *Sacred Sex, A Spiritual Celebration of Oneness in Marriage*, p. 137
30 On behalf of the Universal House of Justice, *Lights of Guidance*, #1226
31 Sue Johnson, Clinical Psychologist, *Hold Me Tight, Seven Conversations for a Lifetime of Love*, p. 186
32 'Abdu'l-Bahá, *Tablets of Abdu'l-Bahá*, Vol. 3, pp. 605-606
33 William J. Doherty, PhD, *Take Back Your Marriage*, p. 48; p. 50; p. 59
34 'Abdu'l-Bahá, *Promulgation of Universal Peace*, p. 168
35 Stephen M. R. Covey, *Speed of Trust*, p. 220
36 Bahá'u'lláh, *Tablets of Bahá'u'lláh*, p. 26
37 Rúhíyyih Rabbani, *Prescription for Living*, 2nd ed., p. 109
38 N. Jenkins, S. Stanley, W. Bailey, and H. Markman, *You Paid How Much for That?!*, p. 26; pp. 156-159
39 On behalf of Shoghi Effendi, *Lights of Guidance*, #421
40 Universal House of Justice, "Individual Rights and Freedoms", p. 16
41 Susan Heitler, PhD, *Power of Two*, p. 7
42 J. Gottman, C. Notarius, J. Gonso, and H. Markman, *A Couple's Guide to Communication*, pp. 1-2
43 Howard Colby Ives, *Portals to Freedom*, pp. 194-195
44 Shoghi Effendi, *Lights of Guidance*, #291
45 Sandra Gray Bender, PhD, *Recreating Marriage with the Same Old Spouse*; p. 111
46 Marshall B. Rosenberg, PhD, *Nonviolent Communication: A Language of Life*, 2nd ed., p. 49
47 'Abdu'l-Bahá, *Promulgation of Universal Peace*, p. 60, #12
48 On behalf of the Universal House of Justice, *Compilations of Compilations, Vol. II*, #2341
49 Susan Heitler, PhD, *Power of Two, Secrets to a Strong & Loving Marriage*, p. 11
50 Howard Colby Ives, *Portals to Freedom*, p. 120, recalling the words of 'Abdu'l-Bahá when imprisoned with many others in the Holy Land
51 On behalf of the Universal House of Justice to an individual, quoted in a Bahá'í World Centre Research Department Memorandum, January 12, 1997, "The Humorist"
52 Rev. Susan Sparks, *Laugh Your Way to Grace—Reclaiming the Spiritual Power of Humor*, pp. 9-10

53 On behalf of the Universal House of Justice, *Compilation of Compilations, Vol. I*, p. 68, #1.3
54 Howard Colby Ives, *Portals to Freedom*, p. 13
55 'Abdu'l-Bahá, *Foundations of World Unity*, p. 20
56 Arthur Koestler, *The Act of Creation*, Book 1, Part 2, Ch. 7
57 Janet A. Khan, *Prophet's Daughter*, p. 245
58 Stephen Post, *Why Good Things Happen to Good People*, p. 104
59 Stephen Post, *Why Good Things Happen to Good People*, p. 114
60 Universal House of Justice, *Framework for Action*, #33.7
61 On behalf of the Universal House of Justice quoted in the "Understanding Tests" memorandum from the Research Department to the Universal House of Justice, July 17, 1989
62 'Abdu'l-Bahá, *Paris Talks*, p. 112
63 Linda Kavelin Popov, *A Pace of Grace*, p. 93
64 Universal House of Justice, *Framework for Action*, #34.2
65 Raymond Switzer, *Conscious Courtship*, p. 68
66 'Abdu'l-Bahá, *Selections from the Writings of 'Abdu'l-Bahá*, #221
67 Raymond and Furugh Switzer, *Mindful Marriage*, p. 259
68 'Abdu'l-Bahá, *Promulgation of Universal Peace*, p. 375

*Couples are like two wings of a bird—both must be strong partners with equal voices for them to soar!*

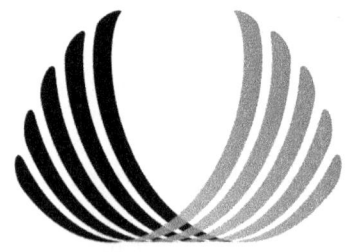

www.marriagetransformation.com
susanne@marriagetransformation.com

www.ingramcontent.com/pod-product-compliance
Lightning Source LLC
Chambersburg PA
CBHW070033040426
42333CB00040B/1582